AF736855

INFECTIONS IN THE IMMUNOCOMPROMISED HOST

Laboratory Diagnosis and Treatment

ADVANCES IN EXPERIMENTAL MEDICINE AND BIOLOGY

Editorial Board:

NATHAN BACK, *State University of New York at Buffalo*

NICHOLAS R. DI LUZIO, *Tulane University School of Medicine*

EPHRAIM KATCHALSKI-KATZIR, *The Weizmann Institute of Science*

DAVID KRITCHEVSKY, *Wistar Institute*

ABEL LAJTHA, *Rockland Research Institute*

RODOLFO PAOLETTI, *University of Milan*

Recent Volumes in this Series

Volume 196
STEROID HORMONE RESISTANCE: Mechanisms and Clinical Aspects
Edited by George P. Chrousos, D. Lynn Loriaux, and Mortimer B. Lipsett

Volume 197
BIOLOGICAL REACTIVE INTERMEDIATES III: Mechanisms of Action in Animal Models and Human Disease
Edited by James J. Kocsis, David J. Jollow, Charlotte M. Witmer, Judd O. Nelson, and Robert Snyder

Volume 198A
KININS IV, Part A
Edited by Lowell M. Greenbaum and Harry S. Margolius

Volume 198B
KININS IV, Part B
Edited by Lowell M. Greenbaum and Harry S. Margolius

Volume 199
NUTRITIONAL AND TOXICOLOGICAL SIGNIFICANCE OF ENZYME INHIBITORS IN FOODS
Edited by Mendel Friedman

Volume 200
OXYGEN TRANSPORT TO TISSUE VIII
Edited by Ian S. Longmuir

Volume 201
LIPOPROTEIN DEFICIENCY SYNDROMES
Edited by Aubie Angel and Jiri Frohlich

Volume 202
INFECTIONS IN THE IMMUNOCOMPROMISED HOST
Laboratory Diagnosis and Treatment
Edited by Paul Actor, Alan Evangelista, James Poupard, and Eileen Hinks

---

A Continuation Order Plan is available for this series. A continuation order will bring delivery of each new volume immediately upon publication. Volumes are billed only upon actual shipment. For further information please contact the publisher.

INFECTIONS IN THE IMMUNOCOMPROMISED HOST

Laboratory Diagnosis and Treatment

Edited by

Paul Actor

Smith Kline and French Laboratories
Philadelphia, Pennsylvania

Alan Evangelista

Cooper Hospital
University Medical Center
Camden, New Jersey

James Poupard

Bryn Mawr Hospital
Bryn Mawr, Pennsylvania

and

Eileen Hinks

Rolling Hill Hospital
Elkins Park, Pennsylvania

PLENUM PRESS • NEW YORK AND LONDON

Library of Congress Cataloging in Publication Data

Eastern Pennsylvania Branch of the American Society for Microbiology Symposium on Infections in the Compromised Host: Laboratory Diagnosis and Treatment: (1983: Philadelphia, Pa.)
Infections in the immunocompromosed host.

(Advances in experimental medicine and biology; v. 202)
"Proceedings of the Eastern Pennsylvania Branch of the American Society for Microbiology Symposium on Infections in the Compromised Host: Laboratory Diagnosis and Treatment, held November 17–18, 1983, in Philadelphia, Pennsylvania"—T.p. verso.
Includes bibliographies and index.
1. Immunological deficiency syndromes—Complications and sequelae—Congresses. 2. Communicable diseases—Congresses. 3. Infection—Congresses. I. Actor, Paul. II. American Society for Microbiology. Eastern Pennsylvania Branch. III. Title. IV. Series. [DNLM: 1. Immunologic Deficiency Syndromes—complications—congresses. 2. Infection—immunology—congresses. W1 AD559/QW 700 E13i 1983]
RC606.E27 1983 616.97 86-15091

ISBN-13: 978-1-4684-1261-1 e-ISBN-13: 978-1-4684-1259-8
DOI: 10.1007/978-1-4684-1259-8

Proceedings of the Eastern Pennsylvania Branch of the American Society for Microbiology Symposium on Infections in the Compromised Host: Laboratory Diagnosis and Treatment, held November 17–18, 1983, in Philadelphia, Pennsylvania

© 1986 Plenum Press, New York

softcover reprint of the hardcover 1st edition 1986

A Division of Plenum Publishing Corporation
233 Spring Street, New York, N.Y. 10013

All rights reserved

No part of this book may be reproduced, stored in a retrieval system, or transmitted in any form or by any means, electronic, mechanical, photocopying, microfilming, recording, or otherwise, without written permission from the Publisher

PREFACE

The subject matter of this volume, the basis for which was a conference held in Philadelphia which focused on the subject of infections, including their diagnosis and treatment, in immunocompromised individuals. The material is of particular importance today when placed against the background of the rapid spread of acquired immunodeficiency syndrome (AIDS).

The first section dealt with the general subject of the immunocompromised host. Here, reviewed in detail, were the epidemiological and clinical aspects of opportunistic infections in patients with defective immune responses. It is widely acknowledged that infections are a major complication of the neoplastic process. Cancer-bearing patients are more prone to certain kinds of infectious and cancer chemotherapy almost always increases susceptibility to such infections. Depending upon the basic disease process of the cancer, a specific array of infectious diseases can be predicted. Patients altered in thymus-derived lymphocyte populations or mononuclear phagocyte capabilities resulting in defects in cell mediated immunity or delayed hypersensitivity become highly susceptible to certain groups of organisms, whereas, profoundly neutropenic patients usually become infected with different organisms. The types of infections noted are relatively predictable for the type of immune defect, with some variations according to epidemiological factors. Major advances have been made in the early diagnosis and treatment of infectious complications with increasingly effective antimicrobial agents and increasing knowledge of their use. The application of so-called preventive procedures has had limited value to date, including immunotherapy, which appears to hold much promise.

Covered also was the immunomodulatory effects of microorganisms and their products. Infectious agents including bacteria, viruses, fungi and parasites can stimulate the nonspecific proliferation and activation of the immune system or specifically stimulate the antimicrobial immune response resulting in humoral antibody or specific sensitized cells. Various microorganisms and their products, especially those derived from mycobacteria, and other intracellular bacteria, can stimulate nonspecific responses and activate macrophages. The perturbation of the immune response observed during experimental and human infections is well-documented. For the most part, this is brought about by either generalized anergy or a selective deregulation of immune responses. Additionally, bacterial, viral and fungal infections have been shown to cause alterations in macrophage function. Parasites can alter the immune response by enhancing polyclonal antibody responses or inducing excessive number of suppressor cells, which inhibit both specific and non-specific immune responses. Viral infections, in man and animals are known to depress existing immune responses including delayed hypersensitivity. Onchogenic viruses may selectively depress certain immune effector cells. Leukemia viruses, in particular, have been widely studied in regards to their effects on immune parameters. These latter studies have direct relevance to AIDS with the demonstration that a human T-cell virus is the etiological agent.

A wide variety of immunomodulatory agents have been studied experimentally in terms of their ability to reverse immunodeficiency induced by tumor viruses. The immunomodulatory properties of products derived from bacteria, including endotoxins, lipoteichoic acids and exotoxins have been shown to be due to selective effects on certain classes of immunocompetent cells. The interaction of bacteria or their products with macrophages results in the release of immunomodulatory mediators. Induction of small molecular weight substances such as prostaglandins also may occur in response to microorganisms or their products on immune response mechanisms.

Subsequent sessions of the Symposium dealt with laboratory aspects of diagnosis of infectious diseases in compromised patients, as well as the description of various opportunistic infections in such patients. Non-tuberculous mycobacterial species are found in increasing numbers in compromised patients. Among these are *Mycobacterium marinum* and *M. intracellulari*. Various aspects of Herpesvirus infections in immunocompromised hosts were covered in detail as were laboratory diagnosis and treatment. Fungal infections continue to be an important pathogen in immunocompromised patients. The role of *Pneumocystis carinii* and other parasitic infections in compromised hosts was discussed as was *Cryptosporidium*, another protozoan parasite.

The effects of various biologically-active agents and immunostimulants on host immune response were covered in the concluding session. Liposomes and other particulate drug carriers can serve as models for localizing drugs predominantly in the mononuclear phagocytic cells of the reticuloendothelial system. Liposomes containing natural and synthetic immunomodulatory or anti-infective drugs (e.g. amphotericin B) have been shown effective in both animal and human infections as well as in animal tumor systems. The potential utility of this approach is compromised by toxicity problems encountered during extended treatment with liposomes with and without immunomodulators. Impairment of RES function and significant bone marrow pathology has been observed in animals treated i.v. with liposomes. These problems are a serious potential limiting factor in the future development of liposomes as a drug delivery system.

The use of lymphokines and other biological response modifiers in the treatment of cancer was reviewed. Attempts to stimulate immune responses with a variety of non-specific immunomodulators in the form of bacterial extracts, viruses and chemicals have been largely unsuccessful in man. The rapid advances with genetically engineered biological products such as lymphokines and ctyokines and monoclonal antibodies may prove useful for cancer treatment, but here again, early results have not been highly successful. Such agents may act directly on tumor cells and/or stimulate the patient to produce an anti-tumor response.

The topics of infectious disease and malignancy in immunocompromised hosts and the immunological defects underlying such conditions are being examined with greater frequency by many scientists. Cooperative efforts among immunologists, microbiologists, tumor biologists and clinicians in exploring the nature and mechanism of immunodeficiency in various disease states and the types and frequency of infectious diseases in such patients should provide valuable new knowledge in the future for treating and, perhaps, even preventing such diseases.

Paul Actor

Eileen Hinks

Alan Evangelista

James Poupard

ACKNOWLEDGEMENTS

The editors are grateful to the Eastern Pennsylvania Branch of the American Society for Microbiology under whose sponsorships this Conference was held, and to the members of the organizing committee who worked diligently to make the symposium possible.

We would like to acknowledge the support and sponsorship of Temple University School of Medicine, Hahnemann Medical College, Thomas Jefferson Medical College, and the School of Medicine of the University of Pennsylvania.

The Conference would not have been possible without the generous financial support of Smith, Kline and French Laboratories whose contributions we gratefully acknowledge.

Special thanks is offered to Dr. Toby K. Eisenstein, the branch President, for her encouragement and support of this endeavor. The Pennsylvania Department of Health--Bureau of Laboratories generously provided help with mailing and registrations. Thanks and appreciation to Cat Hebert for his assistance in layout, proof-reading and preparation of the camera-ready copy of the manuscripts.

ORGANIZING COMMITTEE

Program Chairman

Paul Actor, Ph.D.
Smith Kline & French Laboratories
Philadelphia, PA

Program Co-Chairmen

Alan Evangelista, Ph.D.
Cooper Hospital/
Univ. Medical Center
Camden, NJ

James Poupard, Ph.D.
Bryn Mawr Hospital
Bryn Mawr, PA

Committee Members

Carl Abramson, Ph.D.
Pennsylvania College of
Podiatric Medicine
Philadelphia, PA

Josephine Bartola, J.D.
Pennsylvania Department of Health
Lionville, PA

Helen R. Buckley, Ph.D.
Temple University School
of Medicine
Philadelphia, PA

Walter Ceglowski, Ph.D.
Temple University School
of Medicine
Philadelphia, PA

Kenneth R. Cundy, Ph.D.
Temple University School
of Medicine
Philadelphia, PA

Toby K. Eisenstein, Ph.D.
Temple Univesity School
of Medicine
Philadelphia, PA

Linda Ann Miller, M.S., M.T.
(A.S.C.P.)
Bryn Mawr Hospital
Bryn Mawr, PA

Louis Nisbet, Ph.D.
Smith Kline & French Labs.
Philadelphia, PA

CONTENTS

THE IMMUNOCOMPROMISED HOST - AN OVERVIEW

BACTERIAL AND VIRAL INFECTIONS IN THE COMPROMISED HOST

FUNGAL AND PARASITIC INFECTIONS IN THE IMMUNOCOMPROMISED HOST - AN OVERVIEW

IMMUNOTHERAPY

EPIDEMIOLOGIC AND CLINICAL ASPECTS OF OPPORTUNISTIC INFECTIONS

Donald Armstrong

Infectious Disease Service of the Department of Medicine
Memorial Sloan-Kettering Cancer Center
New York, New York

INTRODUCTION

Infections in the immunocompromised host occur because of immune defects and epidemiological influences. They are often referred to as opportunistic infections, but many are caused by organisms, such as the pneumococcus, that infect apparently immunologically normal individuals. The infections are usually more severe in the immunocompromised host. There are, in addition, certain organisms such as Pneumocystis carinii that only infect immunocompromised individuals. In this paper, a clinical approach to the immunocompromised host is presented along with some selected features concerning therapy. With the exception of a few general references, the literature cited here reflects our experience at Memorial Sloan-Kettering Cancer Center (MSKCC).

IMMUNE DEFECT

For many years, it has been evident that infections in immunocompromised hosts are on the increase. Recently, international meetings have been devoted to this subject[1,2]. A major example is that of infectious complications of neoplastic disease[3]. The neoplastic disease can make patients more prone to infectious complications and the chemotherapy of the neoplasms almost always make patients more prone to infections. The same is true of a number of other diseases, such as collagen vascular, or some hematologic disorders, such as sickle cell disease. A variety of patterns of infectious disease have emerged according to the type of immunosuppression resulting from the basic disease and its therapy. The patient who is profoundly neutropenic becomes highly susceptible to a certain group of organisms while

Table 1. Immune Defects and Infecting Organisms to be Anticipated in the Immunocompromised Host

Immune Defect	Examples	Bacteria	Fungi	Parasites	Viruses
Interrupted Integument	IV needles catheters Chemotherapy induced G.I. ulcers Finger or bone marrow puncture Bladder catheters	Streptococcus pyogenes Staphylococcus aureus Enterobacteriaceae Pseudomonas aeruginosa Staphylococcus epidermidis Corynebacterium spp. Water borne organisms e.g. Serratia marcescens, Pseudomonads	Candida spp. Mucoraceae Aspergillus		
Infusion Infections	Blood products IV fluids	Salmonella spp. Enterobacter agglomerans Enterobacter cloacae	Candida spp.	Plasmodium spp. Toxoplasma gondii Babesia spp.	Hepatitis B Cytomegalovirus Epstein-Barr virus Hepatitis non A & B AIDS
Surgical Procedures	Tracheostomy Respiratory assistance Endoscopies G.I. or Gyn. surgery	Streptococcus pyogenes Staphylococcus aureus Enterobacteriaceae Pseudomonas aeruginosa Bacteroides fragilis	Candida spp.		

Neutrophil	Acute leukemia Chemotherapy	Streptococcus pyogenes Staphylococcus aureus Enterobacteriaceae Pseudomonas aeruginosa	Candida spp. Aspergillus spp. Mucoraceae Trichosporon spp.		
Lymphocyte	Hodgkin's disease Chemotherapy	Listeria monocytogenes Salmonella spp. Nocardia asteroides Mycobacterium spp. Legionella pneumophila Corynebacterium equi	Cryptococcus neoformans Candida spp. Histoplasma capsulatum Coccidioides immitis	Pneumocystis carinii Toxoplasma gondii Strongyloides stercoralis	Measles Herpes simplex Varicella-zoste Cytomegalovirus Adenovirus
Gamma Globulin	Multiple myeloma Chronic lymphocytic leukemia Chemotherapy	Streptococcus pneumoniae Hemophilus influenzae Enteric bacilli		Pneumocystis carinii Giardia lamblia	Echo virus
Complement	Congenital defects	Neisseria meningitidis			
Spleen	Staging Laparatomy for Hodgkin's disease Post trauma	Streptococcus pneumoniae Hemophilus influenzae Neisseria meningitidis		Babesia spp. Plasmodium spp.	

the patient who is altered in the thymus-derived lymphocyte (T lymphocyte-mononuclear phagocyte arm of the immune reaction (cell-mediated immunity or delayed hypersensitivity) becomes susceptible to a different group of organisms (Table 1). People with hypogammaglobulinemia become susceptible to certain types of infection, but they can be highly specific such as persistent, severe Giardia lamblia infections, as seen in patients with IgA deficiencies. Most patients with hypogammaglobulinemia develop repeated upper and lower respiratory tract infections with oral flora, but especially Streptococcus pneumoniae and Hemophilus influenzae. Individuals who have splenic dysfunction or splenectomies are placed at high risk of severe infection with a more limited number of microorganisms, while people with selected complement defects become more susceptible to Neisseria meningitidis. Observations on these patterns have accumulated over the years showing that they are relatively predictable for the type of immune defect with some variation according to epidemiological factors such as travel, work, or pet contact. Iatrogenic factors such as an interrupted integument or transfusion of blood products also results in predictable infections. A number of centers where there are treatment programs for patients with neoplastic disease have collected data on the epidemiology, prevention, early diagnosis, and treatment of the infections occurring in these patients[1-3]. It has become evident that the major advances have been made in the early diagnosis and prompt treatment of infectious complications with increasingly effective antimicrobial agents and increasing knowledge of how to use them. Preventive means, including immunotherapy, hold promise but still remain experimental and, for the most part, of minor or unproven efficacy.

The alteration in immune response may be due to the basic disease such as absent delayed hypersensitivity reactions seen with Hodgkin's disease, lymphomas or hairy cell leukemia or to inadequate functioning neutrophils due to acute leukemia or chronic granulomatous disease of childhood. Multiple myeloma and chronic lymphatic leukemia are regularly associated with hypogammaglobulinemia, while acquired or congenital hypogammaglobulinemia places the patient at similar risks. Sickle cell disease, because of repeated splenic infarction, results in a relative decrease in splenic function while splenectomy for trauma or staging of Hodgkin's disease results in an absolute absence of splenic function.

The therapy of the underlying disease adds to or, by itself, can create the major immune defect. The most common is neutropenia resulting from cytotoxic therapy, but altered delayed hypersensitivity due to adrenocorticosteroid therapy is also common. Drugs such as prednisone also alter neutrophil function while cytotoxic agents, antimetabolites and radiotherapy affect

T lymphocyte-mononuclear phagocyte function in addition to decreasing neutrophil function and numbers. The defects are not always so isolated as indicated, but usually one predominates over the others.

EPIDEMIOLOGY

The epidemiology of infections in the immunocompromised host generally is dependent on the microbial flora of the patient and the hospital where the patient is treated, either as an inpatient or an outpatient. Other factors, however, may be of paramount importance. Previous residence, travel, work, people and pets at home, and hobbies, all may expose the patient to specific opportunistic infections (Table 2). The only way to ascertain these facts so that these infections can be anticipated is by a detailed, carefully obtained history. This should include all previous hospital records which should be rapidly obtained and carefully reviewed and recorded in the chart.

HOSPITAL EPIDEMIOLOGY

Each hospital has its own microbial flora and this is regularly added to the normal flora of the patient. This includes nasopharynx, small and large bowel, and skin. The gastrointestinal tract may become colonized with hospital-acquired organisms such as *Pseudomonas aeruginosa* or *Klebsiella pneumoniae*. Resistant *Escherichia coli* may also become a part of the patient's normal bowel flora, perhaps as a result of antibiotic pressure and plasmid-transferred resistance from hospital-acquired organisms. Waterborne organisms such as *Serratia marcescens* or pseudomonas may colonize bladder and/or intravenous catheters. *S. marcescens* has been found to grow luxuriantly in unsterilized urinometers left over days in patients' rooms. Hospital-acquired *Staphylococcus aureus* tends to colonize the nasopharynx and *Staphylococcus epidermidis*, the skin, although either may apparently invade from the gastrointestinal tract in neutropenic patients. *Corynebacterium* CDC-JK colonization of the skin of the axillae and groin has been discouraged by rigorous attention to hygiene, namely bathing twice daily with a providine soap. Salmonella sepsis has been transferred through the use of contaminated endoscopes and other hospital outbreaks[4] with *Legionella* species, apparently from a water source, has caused significant infections in renal transplant patients in one hospital and patients with neoplastic disease in another[5]. Urinary tract colonization or infection with relatively sensitive organisms may be supplanted by more resistant hospital-acquired bacteria, especially if the patient's urinary tract is instrumented or indwelling bladder catheters are used.

Table 2. Epidemiological Considerations in Opportunistic Infections

Environment	Examples	Comments
Hospitals		
Bacteria	S. aureus P. aeruginosa K. pneumoniae Serratia marcescens Pseudomonads S. epidermidis Corynebacterium CDC-JK Salmonella spp. Legionella spp.	Organisms vary from hospital to hospital. Some associated with colonization such as enterobacteriaceae and P. aeruginosa and others with procedures such as S. marcescens, and Pseudomonads.
Fungi	Candida albicans Candida tropicalis Candida parapsilosis Aspergillus spp. Mucoraceae	C. parapsilosis associated with TPN, C. tropicalis with neutropenia, Aspergillus flavus with construction.
Parasites	Pneumocystis carinii scabies	Can be prevented by early diagnosis and appropriate isolation techniques.
Viruses	Influenza virus Varicella-zoster Cytomegalovirus	Spread by both aerosolization and contact with secretions and excretions.

(Continued)

Geographic		
Bacteria	M. tuberculosis	More common in Third World countries
Fungi	H. capsulatum C. immitis B. dermatides	More common certain parts of North, Central and S. America. Latent infection.
Parasites	Strongyloides Babesia Malaria	More common in tropics and subtropics. Well known distribution nationally and internationally. May be latent infection.
Viruses	Measles	Still endemic in Third World

Table 2 (Continued)

Home Environment		
Bacteria	M. tuberculosis	Household contacts at high risk
Fungi	Aspergillus spp.	Flourish in moist environments including air conditioners and moisteners
Parasites	Scabies	Children may bring home
Viruses	Varicella-zoster virus Influenza	Home contacts a regular source
Work, Habits & Hobbies		
Bacteria	DF-2 of dogs, Campylobacter	Pets
	L. monocytogenes	Farm animals, pets, raw vegetables
	Corynebacterium equi	Farm animals
	Aeromonas hydrophila	Case attributed to wading without boots while fishing

Table 2 (Continued)

Fungi	H. capsulatum	Chicken coops, birding, spelunking
	B. dermatitidis	dogs harbor?
Parasites	Toxoplasma	Cats, raw meat consumption
	Strongyloides	Walking bare foot
	Scabies	Nursery schools, crowded poor economic Environments, hospitals
	G. lamblia	Outbreaks in ski resorts and certain countries
	Malaria & Babesia	Outdoor recreation increases risk
Viruses	Cytomegalovirus	STD especially among homosexuals
	Herpes simplex	STD

It has become apparent that certain Candida species have a predilection for infecting certain types of hospitalized patients. Candida tropicalis causes invasive infection in neutropenic patients arising either from a gastrointestinal or intravenous catheter source while Candida parapsilosis causes relatively benign intravenous catheter infections in patients receiving total parenteral nutrition. Candida albicans causes both bothersome mucous membrane infection in patients with altered T lymphocyte-mononuclear phagocyte function and invasive infections in patients who are neutropenic or those with intravenous catheters. It is not clear whether these organisms are hospital-acquired. Candida species, Mucoraceae and Aspergillus species have all been implicated in point source hospital-acquired infection in various types of immunocompromised patients[6] including those with extensive burns.

Pneumocystis carinii pneumonia has been observed in clusters in a number of hospitals. Scabies of a particularly severe nature has been observed in immunocompromised hosts and, although it is more likely to infect health care personnel, it can spread to other patients.

Viruses have been implicated in hospital-acquired infections. Influenza virus has been described infecting multiple patients in an intensive care unit and the true incidence may be greater than known since often the diagnosis is usually not considered and documented. Varicella-zoster virus may spread from a patient with herpes zoster and cause life threatening varicella in a susceptible individual, either another patient or health care personnel. The latter individuals could spread the disease during the incubation period. Appropriate precautions should be taken -- we isolate herpes zoster or varicella patients and we attempt to obtain serology on all employees and warn those who are susceptible. If an individual is inadvertently exposed, we reassign them away from patient contact during the period of incubation when they might be contagious.

GEOGRAPHIC CONSIDERATIONS

Past residence or travel may be all important in infections in the immunocompromised host. People from areas of high incidence of tuberculosis such as India, Asia, South and Central America, the Carribean and Africa are more likely to develop recrudescent tuberculosis from a latent source during immunosuppression. This does not mean that we should not be alert to this diagnosis in people from the Western world. Individuals over 45 years old are more likely to have been exposed to tuberculosis and suffer breakdown of latent infections. People who have traveled in endemic areas of Histoplasma capsulatum,

Coccidioides immitis, or *Blastomyces dermatitidis* may have had asymptomatic infections which can become latent and subsequently disseminate during immunospression. These fungi are not only endemic in North America, but also in Central and South America and the Carribean Islands. Residence in areas such as the tropics or subtropics will alert us to possible latent parasitic infections such as Strongyloides and malaria. In addition, there are parasites of temperate zones such as Babesia that we must consider.

HOME ENVIRONMENT

The home environment includes the people living there at present and the people with whom the patient has lived in the past. Family contacts, even in the past, are a frequent source of tuberculosis and children in a family can bring varicella virus infection to a susceptible host. Influenza frequently spreads among family members, and scabies or cytomegalovirus may be brought home from a day care center or school to cause severe infection in an immunocompromised host.

WORK HABITS AND HOBBIES

Different types of work are known to expose individuals to various infections, some of which are opportunistic. Working with animals, both pets and farm animals, exposes individuals to various microorganisms. Dogs harbor a fastidious Gram-negative rod, called DF-2, which has usually infected patients with neutrophil defects. Opportunistic Campylobacter infections have also been attributed to dog contact. *G. lamblia* has passed from infected pet birds to humans. Cats are well known to harbor *Toxoplasma gondii*. *Listeria monocytogenes* has been isolated from farm animals and people working in slaughter houses carry the organism in the gastrointestinal tract more often than the general population. Exposure to *Aspergillus* species and *B. dermatitidis* is frequent among those working with compost, and the soil in chicken coops often yields both *H. capsulatum* and *B. dermatitidis* on culture. Individuals' work or hobbies may take them to outdoor areas as described above or to areas endemic for tropical diseases or even into caves spelunking where *H. capsulatum* may reside in abundance in bat feces. The same organism abounds in the feces of blackbirds which may roost on construction sites or golf courses or in the feces of swallows which may roost in chimneys. The habit of eating rare or raw meat may expose an individual to *T. gondii*, which subsequently can recrudesce causing life-threatening encephalitis in an immunocompromised host. Patients with lymphomas who have had exposure to farm animals have developed life-threatening infections with *Corynebacterium equi* and a leukemic patient who waded in lakes fishing without boots developed Aeromonas hydrophila skin lesions with dissemination.

Cytomegalovirus and herpes simplex are sexually transmitted and more prevalent in promiscuous people and can cause life-threatening infection in immunocompromised hosts. People who wear shoes seldom develop Strongyloides stercoralis infections.

CLINICAL ASPECTS

To illustrate clinical aspects of opportunistic infections in the immunocompromised host, four regional infections will be discussed as well as an approach to fever without evident source.

Central Nervous System Infections

At Memorial Sloan-Kettering Cancer Center (MSKCC), the most common cause of bacterial meningitis has been L. monocytogenes. The second most common cause has been P. aeruginosa. These usually occur in two very different types of immunocompromised hosts (Table 3). Regularly, the type of organism infecting correlates with the immune defect[7]. If the patient has a normal leucocyte count and a disease or therapy affecting T lymphocyte-mononuclear phagocyte function and develops meningitis, the causes in order of frequency will be L. monocytogenes, C. neoformans or S. penumoniae. In contrast, if a neutropenic patient develops meningitis it is far more likely due to P. aeruginosa, E. coli or K. penumoniae. Neutropenic patients developed headache or still neck in only 35% of episodes in one series. Mental changes were present however in 93%[8]. If a neutropenic patient develops a brain abscess, the most likely causes are the same bacteria which produce meningitis plus the Mucoraceae, Aspergillus species or Candida species. In contrast, when a patient with a T lymphocyte-mononuclear phagocyte defect develops a brain abscess, the most likely organisms are T. gondii or N. asteroides. Cryptococcomas or tuberculomas have also been described but are rare.

In the meningitides, the diagnosis is usually straightforward in neutropenic patients. There are ample organisms in most cases. In the patient with L. monocytogenes, the cerebrospinal fluid (CSF) pleocytosis is not specific, either mononuclear cells or neutrophils can predominate, and the organisms are seen on Gram stain in only 10.5% in our experience[9]. With C. neoformans, the organisms were seen in 55% of cases[10], but specific cryptococcal antigen was always present. Thus a patient whose immune defect is predominantly T lymphocyte-mononuclear phagocyte who develops a meningitis and the CSF yields no visible organisms and who has a negative cryptococcal antigen test, should be treated empirically

Table 3. Central Nervous System Infections: Immune Defects and Infecting Organisms to be Anticipated in the Immunocompromised Host

Immune Defect	Bacteria	Fungi	Parasites	Viruses
T Lymphocyte mononuclear phagocyte	Listeria monocytogenes (M) Nocardia asteroides (A) Mycobacterium avium-intracellulare	Cryptococcus neoformans (M)	Toxoplasma (AME) Strongyloides stercoralis (M)	Varicella-zoster (ME) Cytomegalovirus (E)
Neutrophil	Enteric bacilli (M) Pseudomonas aeruginosa (M) Bacillus spp. (M)	Aspergillus spp. (A) Mucoraceae (A) Candida spp. (ME)		
Gamma Globulin	Streptococcus pneumoniae (M)			ECHO virus (ME)
Spleen	Streptococcus pneumoniae (M) Neisseria meningitidis (M)			
Complement	Neisseria meningitidis (M)			

Key: M = meningitis
ME = meningoencephalitis
A = abscess

for L. monocytogenes with ampicillin while awaiting the cultures. If the cryptococcal antigen test is positive, it should be possible to isolate the organisms if enough CSF is obtained--we recommend a minimum of 10 ml. Therapy with amphotericin B after finding a positive antigen and while awaiting cultures is reasonable. It must be stressed that for both L. monocytogenes and C. neoformans, it may be necessary to obtain large amounts (up to 20 ml) of CSF to isolate the microorganisms. S. stercoralis meningitis, occuring usually in patients on high doses of adrenocorticosteroids, is suggested by the isolation of bowel flora from the CSF of such an immunocompromised host. One of our patients had P. aeurginosa, enterococcus and C. albicans in the CSF along with S. stercoralis. These same organisms were isolated from the blood before they appeared in the CSF. In this type of clinical setting, polymicrobic sepsis should suggest the diagnosis of the hyperinfection syndrome due to S. stercoralis.

Varicella-zoster virus encephalitis occurs in the setting of severe varicella or disseminated herpes zoster. Treatment with adenosine arabinoside or acyclovir should be instituted in this setting. The virus has only rarely been isolated from the CSF.

Cytomegalovirus has been isolated from the brains of patients with AIDS and an encephalitis. Its role in the encephalitis remains uncertain. There is no effective treatment. Likewise, Mycobacterium avium-intracellulare has been isolated from the brains of AIDS patients at autopsy, but its role in CNS disease is uncertain. Treatment is outlined under gastrointestinal infections. Toxoplasma encephalitis requires sulfadiazine and pyrimethamine, and although treatment of patients with this infection complicating neoplastic disease has not been very effective[11], better results have been seen in AIDS patients with T. gondii encephalitis, although prolonged (3 to 6 months) therapy seems necessary to prevent relapse[12]. N. asteroides brain abscess requires 4 to 6 months of sulfadiazine or cotrimoxazole and drainage or extirpation of large available lesions seems advisable.

Splenectomized patients, especially those with an underlying disease such as Hodgkin's disease, may develop rapidly fatal pneumococcal meningitis. The pneumococcal vaccine has not been effective in reliably producing antibody or protecting against meningitis in our experience. Although the vaccine should be given, prophylactic penicillin should also be administered. The duration of penicillin prophylaxis is uncertain.

In patients with complement deficiencies, the meningococcal meningitis usually responds well to penicillin, but repeated episodes suggest an immune defect and complement, as well as gammaglobulin, measurements should be done.

PNEUMONIAS

The major causes of penumonias in the immunocompromised host are listed in Table 4 under the immune defect which they complicate.

A person with a profoundly low neutrophil count will not develop an exuberant inflammatory response in the lung and therefore will not develop clear signs of pneumonia on physical exam. Little or no sputum is produced and pulmonary infiltrates develop slowly on chest roentgenogram. Due to the lack of sputum, empirical antibacterial therapy with a regimen that will effectively treat potential respiratory pathogens such as streptococci, Klebsiella pneumoniae, E. coli and S. aureus are necessary. One such regimen would be cefazolin, ticarcillin, and gentamicin, which should be effective against most of the mentioned bacteria listed above and isolated in our hospital (Table 4).

The fungi listed in Tables 1 and 4, usually invade later in a patient's hospitalization--at least after the first week. Aspergillus species are the most common fungi causing penumonia--and have been associated with construction or inadequately cleaned air conditioners in hospitals. Sputums are usually negative in patients with invasive disease (66% in a recent series) and positive sputums may represent colonization only[13]. There are serological tests for antibody which are positive in up to 70% of cases, but serum specimens must be collected serially and prospectively to make an early diagnosis[13,14]. A test for circulating antigen has also appeared promising[15]. Lung biopsy may be necessary to differentiate between bacterial or Aspergillus species pneumonia in this clinical setting, but more and more patients are being treated empirically and biopsies postponed to see if there is a response to amphotericin B. If there is no response, then a biopsy is considered, but in some cases it may be too late to perform such an invasive procedure. Responses to amphotericin B are often seen but cure is almost invariably associated with remissions in the neoplastic disease. Pneumonias due to Mucoraceae have not been diagnosed by sputum studies or serology. Biopsies have been necessary. The lesions on x-ray resemble aspergillosis so that empirical therapy with amphotericin B may be administered based on that diagnosis. Since amphotericin B is the treatment of choice for the Mucoraceae, we may not make a specific diagnosis if the patient goes into remission and responds. If the patient relapses and has to receive further chemotherapy and is anticipated to have prolonged neutropenia, then amphotericin B should be considered during chemotherapy to prevent recurrence of aspergillosis and mucormycosis, both of which tend to recur. If there are single pulmonary lesions, some of our hematologists

Table 4. Pneumonias: Immune Defects and Organisms to be Anticipated in the Immunocompromised Host

Immune Defect	Bacteria	Fungi	Parasite	Viruses
Neutrophil	Streptococcus pneumoniae Streptococcus pyogenes Staphylococcus aureus Klebsiella pneumoniae Escherichia coli Other Enterobacteriaceae Pseudomonas aeruginosa Bacillus spp.	Aspergillus spp. Mucor spp. Candida spp.		
T lymphocyte mononuclear phagocyte	Nocardia asteroides Legionella spp. Mycobacteria spp. Corynebacterium spp. Chlamydiae	Cryptococcus neoformans Histoplasma capsulatum Coccidioides immitis Blastomyces	Pneumocystis carinii Toxoplasma gondii Strongyloides stercoralis	Cytomegalovirus Varicella-zoster Adenovirus Measles
Gamma Globulin	Streptococcus pneumoniae Hemophilus influenzae		Pneumocystis carinii	
Spleen	Streptococcus pneumoniae Hemophilus influenzae			Varicella-zoster

prefer to have them surgically removed during remission. Candida species rarely cause a primary pneumonia[16]. They may reach the lung via the hematogenous route when dissemination occurs and then appear as multiple, bilateral, small nodules. Sputum studies yield predominately false-positive results in the colonized high risk patients, but false-negative results have also been recorded. Tests for antibody, antigen, and metabolites of Candida species are discussed under intraabdominal infections. Our patients with Candida pneumonia have had elevated arabinitol/creatinine ratios. Treatment is amphotericin B. the addition of 5-fluorocytosine (flucytosine) may improve chances for recovery, especially if the infection is due to C. tropicalis[17].

In patients with a T lymphocyte-mononuclear phagocyte defect, the pulmonary infections to be anticipated are very different. Nocardia asteroides usually produces dense pulmonary infiltrates, which can go on to cavitation, but rarely, a diffuse pneumonia is seen. Skin lesions may occur which afford the clinician the opportunity to make a rapid diagnosis by aspiration or biopsy. Multiple sputum may be necessary before the organisms are seen or isolated[18] and the laboratory should be advised that N. asteroides is under consideration so that a prolonged search of smears can be done and cultures held for 5 days or more to allow time for the slow-growing colonies to appear. The organisms, when present, take the Gram stain well and modified acid fast stains should not displace careful searching of the Gram stain. Treatment is described under CNS infections.

Legionella species penumonias can be diagnosed by a direct fluorescent antibody (DFA) test, but false negative results are common. Since antibody titers rise only after 2 to 4 weeks of illness, empirical therapy is usually necessary and should be instituted even in the face of a negative direct fluorescent antibody smear if the clinician is sufficiently suspicious of legionellosis. Erythromycin should be started at 60 mgms/kgm/day in 4 divided doses and after a week it can be reduced to 30 mgm/kgm/day.

Pulmonary disease due to M. tuberculosis can be diagnosed only if appropriate stains and cultures are done. It also may progress very rapidly and resemble an acute pyogenic pneumonia in these patients. It may be more subacute and resemble Nocardiosis. Controlled studies are not available and are not likely to become available, but it seems prudent to start therapy with INH and rifampin and one other drug such as ethambutol or streptomycin. Atypical mycobacterioses also require appropriate smears and cultures. If strongly suspected, for example in and AIDS patients, the clinician should not wait for identification and sensitivities. Empirical therapy should be started. At the least this would mean giving INH, ethambutol, ansamycin, clofazamine, and ethionamide to cover M. tuberculosis and M. avium-intracellulare.

Corynebacterium equi has rarely been implicated in pneumonia in lymphoma patients. Skin lesions may yield the isolate as well as might blood and sputum cultures[19]. the laboratory must recognize the isolate in the sputum as not just another Corynebacterium species. When treated, it has responded to erythromycin. Chlamydiae have caused pneumonias in children with severe combined immunodeficiency syndrome (SCID). The species implicated, C. trachomatis, should be seen on routine iodine stains of inoculated cell cultures, but C. psittaci, another possible candidate, is recognized by Giemsa stain. This stain should also be used on biopsy or autopsy specimens. Both Chlamydia species may cause respiratory disease in immunocompromised hosts more than we realize.

The fungi causing pneumonias usually do so as part of a disseminated infection. C. neoformans will occasionally present as a pneumonia rather than meningitis. Sputums are not regularly positive. Antigen has been detected in the blood of such patients[20]. Treatment should be with Amphotericin B and flucytosine. H. capsulatum[6] may cause mediastinal lymphadenopathy along with the pneumonia, and skin lesions may also appear. The diagnosis is most readily made by bone marrow aspiration and biopsy and culture. Serology is usually not helpful. Amphotericin B is the initial treatment of choice, ketoconazole may be used later after response is evident and the patient can be switched to an oral drug. Recurrence has been a problem with ketoconazole therapy. Coccidioides immitis may also cause a pneumonia, along with meningitis. Isolation of the organism from sputum or even CSF may be difficult. Serology is frequently helpful and should be performed. If a delay is to be expected, therapy with amphotericin B should be started empirically. Ketoconazole may then subsequently be used. Blastomycosis is the least commonly occurring of the opportunistic fungi, but when it occurs pneumonias are prominent. The budding yeasts with "thick necks" and small double capsules are evident on wet mount of the sputum. Skin or bone lesions may yield the organism on biopsy. Amphotericin B is the treatment of choice.

Among the parasites, P. carinii is the most common cause of opportunistic pneumonia. It is the most common infection recognized antemortem in AIDS patients. The most efficient method of diagnosis is a bronchoalveolar lavage[21] and a number of stains are available to the microbiologist such as the Gram-Wiegart or Toluidine blue for cysts or Giemsa for trophozoites in addition to the methenamine silver stain done by pathologists. Cultures for cytomegalovirus should also be done because it often is found in association with P. carinii. AIDS patients do poorly when they have such dual pneumonias. A transbronchial biopsy or, less often, sputum cytology, can reveal typical "Owls Eye" inclusions of CMV.

Toxoplasma gondii rarely causes pneumonia in immunocompromised patients with T cell defects. It more often causes encephalitis. Lung biopsy or serology is necessary for the diagnosis. Treatment has been discussed under CNS infections. Strongyloides stercoralis is also a rare cause of pneumonia in such patients and the clinical presentation has been discussed under CNS infections.

Cytomegalovirus pneumonia has been briefly discussed above. It mimics P. carinii pneumonia appearing as an acute diffuse process with both interstitial and alveolar components. It may be slowly or rapidly progressive. Diagnosis should be made by biopsy or cytology done on bronchoalveolar lavage, although experience with the latter is more limited. There is presently no specific therapy. Prevention using either interferon or hyperimmune globulin in high risk individuals, such as renal or bone marrow transplant patients, seems promising.

Varicella-zoster virus pneumonia is usually clinically evident because the typical rash is present. A lung biopsy is seldom necessary unless a concomitant infection is strongly suspected. Adenosine arabinoside was the treatment of choice, although acyclovir appears to be equally effective.

Adenovirus pneumonias have been observed in bone marrow transplant patients and appeared to have contributed significantly to the patients' death. The isolates have been, in addition to the more common serotypes, type 34 and 35, similar to the isolates from AIDS patients. Open lung biopsy seems the only effective method of diagnosis. There is no treatment. Measles virus has caused a severe giant cell pneumonia in children with acute lymphocytic leukemia, but this has not been seen in recent years.

Hypogammaglobulinemic individuals suffer repeated episodes of pneumococcal pneumonia. This may alternate with episodes of H. influenzae pneumonia especially if the patient has developed chronic lung disease with bronchiectasis. Pooled gammaglobulin inoculations are frequently administered and do seem to decrease the number of episodes in patients with congenital or acquired hypogammaglobulinemia. Intravenous gammaglobulin seems even more promising. This is not so clear in people with secondary hypogammaglobulinemia due to multiple myeloma or chronic lymphatic leukemia. Acute pneumonias seem more common in these patients. Splenectomy also makes patients prone to pneumococcal, Hemophilus, and meningococcal infections, but with the former, sepsis without evident source and spread to the meninges is more common.

P. carinii pneumonia has occurred in children with congenital immune deficiencies manifested primarily by hypogammaglobulinemia, but combined immune deficiencies were not ruled out. A rare case in a patient with multiple myeloma might also be attributed to prolonged chemotherapy altering the T lymphocyte-mononuclear phagocyte function.

Intraabdominal and Gastrointestinal Infections

The most common source for sepsis in the neutropenic host appears to be the gastrointestinal tract, either the large or small bowel. Clinically, the source is inapparent and we have learned through postmortem examinations that microorganisms normally (or hospital-acquired) residing in the bowel invade through ulcers that we assume have been caused by chemotherapeutic agents. In the absence of neutrophils, and also of platelets, the Enterobacteriaceae, P. aeruginosa, and other organisms such as Aeromonas hydrophila can invade and disseminate (Table 5). The order of frequency of bloodstream invasion correlates well with the numbers of each type of organism residing in the bowel either naturally or as a result of colonization of hospital-acquired organisms or influenced by antibiotic pressure. E. coli and K. pneumoniae are most common early in the hospital course followed by P. aeruginosa, Enterobacter species, and Candida species. S. aureus and even S. epidermidis also seem to be invading from this source. Sometimes the source of entry is apparent if it is the mouth, esophagus, or an anorectal lesion, but more often it is in a site that does not cause symptoms or signs. The typical picture is that the neutropenic patient develops fever, looks toxic, and on history and physical exam there is no obvious source for the fever. We have learned to treat empirically--and early--with an antibiotic regimen to cover the most likely causes of sepsis from the bowel (Table 6). In addition, Clostridum species invade from the bowel in neutropenic patients and in patients with necrotic tumor of the bowel. There is a classical clostridial sepsis syndrome that occured in 29% of patients in our experience[22]. The patient is alert, despite hypotension. There is a pulse/temperature discrepancy in that the pulse is more rapid than would be expected from the temperature. When this occurs it is striking and the prognosis is grave because the patient is hemolyzing, which is responsible for the extremely rapid pulse. Early recognition of the syndrome, including aspiration and Gram stain of areas of cellulitis and addition of high dose penicillin to the antibiotic regimen appears important. The mortality from Clostridial isolates is sepsis from the bowel in the neutropenic patient in most cases. In severe cases the organism can be seen on Gram stain of a peripheral blood smear.

Candida species, especially C. albicans and C. tropicalis, invade from the ulcerated bowel in the neutropenic host and this

Table 5. Intraabdominal and Gastrointestinal Infections: Immune Defects and Organisms to be Anticipated in the Immunocompromised Host

Immune Defect	Bacteria	Fungi	Parasite	Viruses
Neutrophil	Enterobacteriaceae Pseudomonas aeruginosa Aeromonas hydrophila Staphylococcus epidermidis Clostridium spp	Candida spp. Aspergillus spp. Mucoraceae Trichosporon spp.		
T lymphocyte mononuclear phagocyte	Salmonella spp. Mycobacterium avium-intracellulare		Strongyloides stercoralis Cryptosporidium spp Isopera belli	Cytomegalovirus Adenovirus
Gamma Globulin			Giardia	ECHO virus

Table 6. Antibiotics for Clinical Sepsis

Immune Defect	
Neutrophil	ticarcillin[+] and gentamicin[++]
	cefazolin, ticarcillin and gentamicin
	oxacillin, ticarcillin and gentamicin
	cefazolin and ticarcillin
	co-trimoxazole and gentamicin
T lymphocyte mononuclear phagocyte	When clinically appropriate defer antibiotics and investigate
	cefazolin and gentamicin
	co-trimoxazole and gentamicin
Interrupted Integument	Remove catheter or drain lesion
	vancomycin and gentamicin
	cefazolin and gentamicin
Splenic dysfunction	penicillin

[+]ticarcillin, piperacillin, azlocillin, mezlocillin may be used interchangeably

[++]tobramycin, amikacin or netilmicin may be used if gentamicin resistance is prevalent

is probably the most common source of candidemia along with intravenous catheter-associated infections. When Candida invades from the gastrointestinal tract there is no distinctive diagnostic feature. When esophagitis is symptomatic and apparent on barium swallow, this does not mean that is due to Candida. Herpes simplex and bacteria can also cause esophagitis and esophagoscopy should be avoided because life-threatening bacteremias have followed this procedure. Blood cultures in invasive candidiasis are positive in only about 50% of cases and they are positive late-reflected by a mortality as high as 90%[17,24,25]. A blood culture system employing direct inoculation onto agar plates has increased the yield by 30%[26], but an earlier diagnosis is clearly necessary. Antibody studies are not effective in most immunocompromised hosts at risk[27]. Antigen detection, using various techniques, has been accurate in carefully controlled studies in about 50% of cases with relatively few false positive results[28,29,30,31]. There have been no studies to demonstrate that therapy based on antigen detection makes a difference. Biochemical determinations of yeast cell constituents or metabolites have been investigated. The use of mannan or mannose levels determined by gas liquid chromatography[32] has yielded different results in different laboratories and is confounded by very variable levels of endogenous mannose. Arabinitol, a polyol, found in large concentrations in most Candida species and also released from the organism during both life and death, can be detected by GLC or mass spectroscopy[33,34,35]. Only low levels are found in normal humans, but levels rise, in direct[36] proportion to creatinine levels, in renal failure. An arabinitol/creatinine (A/C) ratio corrects for this[37] and in one study, 64% of patients with invasive candidiasis had elevated arabinitol levels or arabinitol/creatinine ratios[38]. This was a retrospective study and the influence of A/C ratios on therapeutic intervention has not been determined. It is apparent that a heavy infection is necessary to increase the A/C ratio in an animal model and separation of D-arabinitol produced by the yeasts from L-arabinitol produced by humans should make this test more sensitive and specific. Presently, there is no sensitive and specific test proven efficacious in the early diagnosis of candidiasis. The clinician must put history, physical and laboratory evidence together and then make a clinical decision whether to treat or not for presumptive candidiasis. Most clinicians are treating earlier, rather than later; for instance, amphotericin B is started empirically 5 to 10 days after antibacterial therapy has apparently failed.

Aspergillus species and Mucoraceae rarely invade from the bowel. A diagnosis would have to be made by biopsy. Treatment might include extirpation of the lesion as well as amphotericin B. In some Trichosporon species infections in neutropenic patients, organisms have been found in the bowel where it appeared to be the source. Diagnoses have usually been made from blood cultures or from skin lesions. Trichosporon cutaneum has been resistant to amphotericin B in vitro and sensitive to miconazole. The only patient recovering from trichosporosis, however, was under treatment with amphotericin B when his leukemia went into remission.

T lymphocyte-mononuclear phagocyte defects complicated by intraabdominal infections are caused by the microorganisms listed in Table 5. Salmonellosis with Salmonella serotypes other than typhimurium produce a typhoidal syndrome in 70% of patients with leukemias and lymphomas while enteritis is more common in patients with solid tumors just as it is in the general population. AIDS patients also develop a typhoidal syndrome due to non-typhi serotypes and they also tend to recur after treatment courses of ordinary duration. Shigellosis also tends to recur in these patients.

Mycobacterium avium-intracellulare causes one of the most striking infections seen in AIDS. The patients present with periodic, recurrent diarrhea consisting of 3 to 4 loose stools per day associated with crampy abdominal pain and persistent weight loss. Some patients have had documented malabsorption and on bowel biopsy, a histopathological picture resembling Whipples' Disease. The PAS-positive foamy macrophages, however, are packed with acid fast bacilli which are M. avium-intracellulare. Massive infiltration of lymph nodes and the omentum is common. The liver is often involved. Bacteremias with colony counts as high as 28,000 cfu per ml of blood have been documented[39]. Biopsy of the bowel is the definitive method of diagnosis, but positive AFB smears and cultures of the stool and blood cultures have accompanied the bowel involvement in most cases. Treatment with ansamycin, clofazamine, ethambutol and ethionamide has resulted in decreases in colonly counts in blood, but has had little apparent effect on the M. avium-intracellulare infiltration of the bowel or other organs. In our experience the mycobacterial infections have often been accompanied by disseminated cytomegalovirus infection.

Another extraordinary gastrointestinal infection seen in patients with AIDS is cryptosporidiosis. This had previously been seen as a self-limited, mild to moderately severe, diarrheal disease in veterinarians exposed to infected animals, or a persistent, moderately severe disease in people with hypogammaglobulinemia or severe combined immunodeficiency syndrome. Since the AIDS epidemic, it has been observed causing a persistent, severe cholera-like illness which is readily diagnosed by stool wet mounts, sucrose flotation or acid fast stains on the stools. There is no treatment which has proven consistently efficacious. Some AIDS patients with a mild form have cleared spontaneously. Isospora belli has also caused self-limited infection in normals and AIDS patients and its natural history in the latter is not as yet known.

Strongyloides stercoralis hyperinfection syndrome has been mentioned under CNS and pulmonary infections. During the hyperinfection syndrome a pre-existing eosinophilia regularly disappears. The larvae may only be found in the duodenum early in the infection by doing a "string test". Treatment is with thiabendazole for 5 to 10 days at least, not for the recommended two days for luminal infestations.

Cytomegalovirus infections of the gastrointestinal tract causing colitis are uncommon in most immunocompromised hosts, but are common in AIDS patients. In such patients, the virus often causes severe hepatitis and even adrenalitis with adrenal insufficiency. Diagnosis is by biopsy documenting tissue invasion. Since the virus can colonize and be excreted in the stool without causing invasive disease. There is no treatment. Adenoviruses, especially types 34 and 35, are often found in stools of AIDS patients, but invasive disease appears rare and would have to be documented by histopathology. There is no treatment.

Giardia lamblia and ECHO viruses cause persistent infections in patients with IgA deficiencies. This may be true of cryptosporidia.

Skin Infections

A list of the more commonly seen skin infections according to the immune defect is contained in Table 6. The only organism that produces a clinical picture which is clear-cut is varicella-zoster virus. Rarely, a patch of Herpes simplex lesions may imitate a patch of lesions seen early in herpes zoster. If it is herpes simplex, a culture should yield the organism in 24 to 48 hours. Immunoperoxidase staining may detect antigen in cells even earlier. During that time the other lesions of herpes zoster will usually appear. Varicella (chicken pox) in immunocompromised children may be atypical, especially if low platelet counts promote bleeding into the lesions.

All other skin lesions are not characteristic enough to allow the clinician to make a diagnosis by just examining them. An aspirate or biopsy or both should be done immediately. It may be the only method of making a rapid diagnosis especially in the fungal infections where blood cultures are so often negative and other cultures are misleading because of frequent false positive (e.g., Candida species) or false negative (e.g., Aspergillus species) results. When a clinican sees a skin lesion in an

Table 7. Skin Infections: Immune Defects and Organisms to be Anticipated in the Immunocompromised Host

Immune Defect	Bacteria	Fungi	Parasites	Viruses
Neutrophil	Enterobacteriaceae Pseudomonas aeruginosa Aeromonas hydrophila Mycobacterium Species	Candida spp. Aspergillus spp. Mucoraceae Trichosporon spp.		
T-lymphocyte mononuclear phagocyte	Nocardia asteroides Corynebacterium equi Chromobacterium violaceum	Cryptococcus neoformans Histoplasma capsulatum Blastomyces dermatitidis Candida spp.	Toxoplasma gondii	Varicella-zoster Cytomegalovirus Herpes simplex Adenovirus Measles

immunocompromised host, the immediate reaction should be to aspirate twice--one for smear and one for culture; and if the smear is unrevealing, biopsy twice, one for smear and histopathology and the other for culture.

Clinical Sepsis

Clinical sepsis without an evident source in the neutropenic patient can be caused by a number of organisms (Table 1) usually residing in the gastrointestinal tract. Others such as *Bacillus cereus* or *Bacillus subtilis*, *Capnocytophaga* species or a variety of organisms found in the hospital environment are occasionally responsible. In the neutropenic patient who appears septic, cultures should be obtained and empiric therapy should be used and various regimens are outlined (Table 6). Most regimens include an antipseudomonas penicillin, such as ticarcillin or piperacillin, and an aminoglycoside, such as gentamicin, tobramycin or amikacin. It appears as if using a combination of ticarcillin and gentamicin or its equivalent is equal to the other regimens. The aminoglycoside appears to be sufficiently effective against *S. aureus* to control it until cultures become positive and a semi-synthetic penicillin such as oxacillin can be used. In a hospital where *K. pneumoniae* infections are common, there would be a theoretical advantage to including a cephalosporin with the aminoglycoside, but this has not been documented in controlled studies. The claimed disadvantage of more renal toxicity with a cephalosporin in combination with an aminoglycoside is controversial. The role of second generation cephalosporins is not clear. The role of third generation cephalosporins as single agents or in combination also remains unestablished. Two beta-lactam antibiotics have been used and appear about as effective as regimens containing an aminoglycoside. Many clinicians prefer using an aminoglycoside to achieve synergy with the antipseudomonas penicillin against *P. aeruginosa*. Splenectomized patients should also receive empiric therapy, including penicillin, after appropriate cultures are obtained. In patients with other immune defects, such as an interrupted integument or altered delayed hypersensitivity, time may be available to investigate possible causes. This has to be individualized for each patient. After the antbiotics are started, if the neutropenic patient responds with defervescence and a source or organism is not determined then it must be decided when to stop the antibiotics. As a result of one controlled study it has been suggested that the antibiotics should be continued until the neutrophil count returns to functional levels. It should be noted that this was done on a pediatric service and it is not stated how soon after defervescence antibiotics were stopped[40]. The recommendation from this study, therefore, cannot be generally applied. One method is to stop antibiotics one at a time, 24-28 hours apart starting 3 to 5 days after defervescence, with the last antibiotic to be stopped being the aminoglycoside. Patients would then receive a minimum of 5 days of antibiotics after the fever stopped. In contrast, if the neutropenic patient's temperature does not respond, then antibiotics can be continued, changed, or amphotericin B added. If the febrile patient is not obviously deteriorating, then it can be assumed that, in the presence of neutropenia, the antibiotics are suppressing but not curing the infection, so that change is not always necessary. If bacterial superinfection is considered, then a change in antibiotics should be according to the predominant type of resistant organisms seen in that hospital. For instance, we anticipate superinfection with *Corynebacterium species* CDC-JK or *S. epidermidis* and consider adding vancomycin. There is no definite answer to the question as to when to add amphotericin B. Pulmonary lesions suggest aspergillosis, while eyeground or skin lesions suggest candidiasis, but frequently there are no helpful signs or symptoms and the clinician must make the decision on an individual basis. Definitive laboratory tests are infrequently available or only late. When the decision to add amphotericin B is made, therapeutic doses should be attained within 24 hours. One regimen is as follows: A test dose of 1 mgm IV over 2 hours is given and, if tolerated, followed by increments of 5 to 10 mgms q 6 hours to 0.5 1 mgm/kgm/day. At first the drug should be given daily and subsequently, as the patient stabilizes, every other day. If there is an anaphylactoid reaction to the 1 mgm test dose, then it is worth trying a smaller dose because patients, after such a reaction to 1 mgm, have tolerated 0.1 mgm with increasing increments of 0.5 to 5 mgms every 6 hours, with a build-up to 1 mgm/kgm in 48 hours. Synergism of flucytosine with amphotericin B against *Candida* or *Aspergillus* species has not been clinically documented as it has with *Cryptococcus neoformans*. We have found, from retrospective data, that the addition of flucytosine to amphotericin B has significantly decreased the mortality of *Candida tropicalis* infections in fungemic patients[17]. If we use flucytosine with amphotericin B, we administer flucytosine at 100 mgm/kgm/day in 4 divided doses and follow blood levels. If amphotericin B decreases renal excretion, then flucytosine levels may become high and toxic and the dose must be adjusted. Serological tests for circulating antigen, cell constituents, and metabolites hold promise for offering a more rapid diagnosis, but they all require confirmation. Approaches using immunological and biochemical methods to make rapid and specific microbial diagnoses of causes of clinical sepsis offer great promise for the future care of such patients.

PROTECTIVE ISOLATION

Studies over the years using protective isolation have varied in their results. The most disappointing results came from carefully controlled studies which show no prolongation of life despite some decrease in infection. Since protected environments are expensive, uncomfortable for both patients and staff and are, at most, of minimal benefit, they should remain experimental and be used in carefully controlled studies. It has been stated that patients who are neutropenic for greater than 3 weeks are those who will benefit from a protected environment[1,2,3].

PROPHYLACTIC ANTIBIOTICS

Just as with protective isolation, studies of both non-absorbable and absorbable prophylactic antibiotics in neutropenic patients have resulted in conflicting data. The regimens frequently cause anorexia, nausea or vomiting. Emergence of resistant organisms has been observed[1,2,3]. Since there is no consistent advantage to their use in neutropenic patients, prophylactic antibiotics should remain experimental and studies scrupulously controlled. In sharp contrast, oral trimethoprim-sulfamethoxazole has proved highly effective in protecting high risk patients (children with acute lymphoblastic leukemia) against *P. carinii* pneumonia[1,2,3].

LEUCOCYTE TRANSFUSIONS

The benefits of leucocyte transfusions are also not clear cut. Dangers are apparent. Further, carefully controlled, studies are indicated. It has been recommended that a documented infection that has not responded to 3 days of appropriate antibiotics is an indication for leucocyte transfusions[1,2,3].

IMMUNOTHERAPY

A pseudomonas vaccine has been tried in a controlled study and found wanting. Although there was some protection against lethal *P. aeruginosa* infections, the patients' lives were not prolonged. A varicella-zoster vaccine does seem promising, and needs further study. Hyperimmune globulin has offered protection against varicella-zoster virus if given early after exposure. A hyperimmune globulin to a common Enterobacteriaceae antigen has been beneficial in one study of sepsis and should be further studied[2]. Various other modalities such as interferon, transfer factor, and thymosin need further investigation[1,2,3].

CONCLUSIONS

In the past twenty years there has been little change in the type of organisms infecting immunocompromised patients. Some, such as *P. carinii*, or cytomegalovirus, appear to be causing infection more frequently but this may be a result of increased ability to recognize the organisms as much as it is an actual increase in incidence. It also may be the result of the presence of more patients with the underlying immune defect whose lives are prolonged by modern methods of managing the underlying disease and more effective antimicrobial therapy. The bacteria causing life-threatening infections in neutropenic patients have remained relatively consistent. In most studies, *E. coli*, *K. pneumoniae* and *P. aeruginosa* continue to lead all the rest with *S. aureus* fourth. The increase in incidence of infections with *Candida* and *Aspergillus* species and the Mucorales over the years probably reflects the increased number of patients who survive prolonged periods of neutropenia due to successful treatment of previously lethal bacterial infection. A few new agents such as *Legionella pneumophilia*, *Corynebacterium* CDC-JK, *Capnocytophaga* species and *Trichosporon cutaneum* have recently been recognized as opportunistic pathogens in a small number of cases but may well have been present previously, but went unrecognized.

The AIDS epidemic has revealed a striking predilection for certain organisms for these patients, e.g., *P. carinii* and *M. avium-intracellulare*. They most closely resemble patients with hairy cell leukemia or those following bone marrow transplantation in their immune defect. In addition, certain activities bring them into frequent contact with other opportunistic pathogens; e.g., cytomegalovirus, and cryptosporidiosis. Pinpointing these defects will greatly advance our knowledge of the immunocompromised host and opportunistic pathogens.

REFERENCES

1. J Verhoef, P.K. Peterson, and P.G. Quie, (Eds.), Infections in the immunocompromised host -- Pathogenesis, Prevention, and therapy, *in* "Developments in Immunology," New York, Elsevier/North Holland Biomedical Press, vol 11 (1983).
2. C.S.F. Easmon and H. Gaya (Eds), "Second International Symposium on Infections in the Immunocompromised Host," Academic Press, Inc., New York (1983).
3. A.E. Brown and D. Armstrong, (Eds.), Controversies in the management of infectious complications of neoplastic disease, *Amer.J. Med.* 76:345-766 (1984).
4. D. Armstrong, Infections in patients with neoplastic disease *in* "Infections in the Immunocompromised Host -- Pathogenesis, Prevention, and Therapy," J. Verhoef, et al., (eds.), pp. 129-158 (1980).

5. R.D. Meyer, Legionnaire's Disease. Aspects of nosocomical infection, in "Controversies in the Management of Infectious Complications of Neoplastic Disease," A.E. Brown and D. Armstrong, eds., Amer. J. Med. 76:657-663 (1984).
6. D. Armstrong, Fungal infections in the compromised host, in "Clinical Approach to Infection in the Compromised Host," R.H. Rubin & L.S. Young, eds., Plenum Medical, New York, pp. 195-288 (1981).
7. D. Armstrong and B. Wong, Central nervous system infections in immunocompromised hosts, Ann. Rev. Med. 33:293-308 (1982).
8. S.A. Lukes, J.B. Posner, S. Nielsen, and D. Armstrong, Bacterial infections of the CNS in neutropenic patients, Neurol. 34:269-275 (1984).
9. M.J. Gersten, F. Ognibene, A. Blevins, and D. Armstrong, Listeria infections and neoplastic disease. An old association, recent observations, In preparation.
10. B.P. Polsky, and D. Armstrong, Cryptococcosis, In preparation
11. T.B. Hakes, and D. Armstrong, Toxoplasmosis: Problems in diagnosis and treatment, Cancer 52:1535-1540 (1983).
12. B. Wong, J.W.M. Gold, A.E. Brown, M. Lange, R. Fried, M. Grieco, D. Mildvan, J. Giron, M.L. Tapper, C.W. Lerner and D. Armstrong, Central nervous system toxoplasmosis in homosexual men and parenteral drug abusers in New York: high incidence of infection and abnormal antibody responses, Ann. Intern. Med. 100:36-42 (1984).
13. B. Fisher, D. Armstrong, B. Yu and J.W.M. Gold, Invasive aspergillos: Progress in early diagnosis and treatment, Amer.J.Med. 71:571-577 (1981).
14. J.C. Schaefer, B. Yu and D. Armstrong, An aspergillus immunodiffusion test in the early diagnosis of aspergillosis in adult leukemia patients, Amer. Rev. Resp. Dis. 113:325-329 (1976).
15. M.H. Weiner, G.H. Talbot, S.L. Gerson, G. Filice and P.A. Cassileth, Antigen detection in the diagnosis of invasive aspergillosis, Ann. Intern. Med. 99:777-782 (1983).
16. H. Mazur, P.P. Rosen, and D. Armstrong, Pulmonary disease caused by Candida species, Amer.J.Med. 63:914-925 (1977).
17. R. Horn, B. Wong, T.E. Kiehn, and D. Armstrong, Fungemia in a cancer hospital: increasing frequency, earlier onset and results of therapy in 188 patients. Submitted for publication.
18. L.S. Young, D. Armstrong, A. Blevins, and P. Lieberman, Nocardia asteroides infection complicating neoplastic disease, Amer.J.Med. 50:356-367 (1971).
19. R. Berg, H. Chmel, J. Mayo and D. Armstrong, Corynebacterium equi infection complicating neoplastic disease, Amer.J.Clin.Pathol. 68:73-77 (1977).

20. B.D. Fisher and D. Armstrong, Cryptococcal interstitial pneumonia: Value of antigen determination, New Engl. J. Med. 97:1440-1441 (1977).
21. D.E. Stover, S.I. Hajdu, M.B., Zaman, M.L. Lange, J.W.M. Gold, and D. Armstrong, Bronchoaveolar lavage and the diagnosis of diffuse pulmonary infiltrates in the immunosuppressed host, Annal. Intern. Med. 101:1-7 (1984).
22. J.W. Wynne and D. Armstrong, Clostridial septicemia, Cancer 29:215-221 (1982).
23. E. Whimbey and D. Armstrong, Bacteremia and fungemia in patients with neoplastic disease. In preparation.
24. F.M. Carpentier, T.E. Kiehn and D. Armstrong, Fungemia in the immunocompromised host: changing patterns, antigenemia, high mortality, Amer.J.Med. 71:363-370 (1981).
25. E. Goldstein and P.D. Hoeprich, Problems in the diagnosis and treatment of systemic candidiasis, J. Infect. Dis. 125:190-193 (1972).
26. T.E. Kiehn, B. Wong, F.F. Edwards and D. Armstrong, Comparative recovery of bacteria and yeasts from lysis-centrifugation and a conventional blood culture system, J.Clin. Microbiol. 18:300-304 (1983).
27. G. Filice, B. Yu and D. Armstrong, Immunodiffusion and agglutination tests for Candida in patients with neoplastic disease: Inconsistent correlation of results with invasive infections, J.Infect.Dis. 135:349-357 (1977).
28. M.H. Weiner and W.J. Young, Mannan antigenemia in the diagnosis of invasive Candida infections, J.Clin.Invest. 58:1045-1053 (1976).
29. F.M. Carpentier and D. Armstrong, Candida antigenemia as detected by passive hemagglutination inhibition in patients with disseminated Candidiasis or Candida colonization, J.Clin.Microbiol. 13:10-14 (1981).
30. M.A. Lew, G.R. Siber, D.M. Donahue, and F. Maiorca, Enhanced detection with an enzyme linked immunosorbent assay of Candida mannan in antibody containing serum after heat extraction, J.Infect. Dis. 145-45-56 (1981).
31. P. Stevens, S. Huang, L.S. Young, and M. Berdischewsky, Detection of Candida antigenemia in human invasive Candidiasis by a new solid phase radioimmunoassay, Infection 8: (Suppl. 3) 5334-5338 (1980).
32. G.G. Miller, M.W. Witwer, A.I. Braude, and C.E. Davis, Rapid identification in man by gas-liquid chromatography, J.Clin.Invest. 54:1236-1240 (1974).
33. E.M. Bernard, K.J. Christiansen, S. Tsang, T.E. Kiehn, and D. Armstrong, Rate of arabinitol production by pathogenic yeast species, J. Clin. Microbiol. 14:189-194 (1981).

34. T.E. Kiehn, E.M. Bernard, J.W.M. Gold and D. Armstrong, Candidiasis: detection by gas-liquid chromatography of D-arabinitol, a fungal metabolite, in human serum, Science 206:577-580 (1979).
35. J. Roboz, R. Susuki, and J.F. Holland, Quantification of arabinitol in serum by selected ion monitoring as a diagnostic technique in invasive Candidiasis, J.Clin. Microbiol. 12:594-602 (1980).
36. B. Wong, E. Bernard, J. Gold, D. Fong and D. Armstrong, The arabinitol appearance rate in laboratory animals and humans: estimation from the arabinitol/creatinine ratio and relevance to the diagnosis of Candiasis, J.Infect.Dis. 146:353-3590 (1982).
37. B. Wong, E.M. Bernard, J.W.M. Gold, A. Silber and D. Armstrong, Increased arabinitol levels in experimental Candidiasis in rats: arabinitol appearance rates, arabinitol/creatinine ratios, and severity of infection, J.Infect.Dis. 146:346-352 (1982).
38. J.W.M. Gold, B. Wong, E.M. Bernard, T.E. Kiehn and D. Armstrong, Serum arabinitol concentrations and arabinitol/creatinine ratios in invasive Candidiasis, J.Infect.Dis. 147:504-514 (1983).
39. B. Wong, F.F. Edwards, T.E. Kiehn, E. Whimbey, H. Donnelly, E.M. Bernard, J.W.M. Gold and D. Armstrong, Continuous high-grade Mycobacterium avium-intracellulare bacteremia in patients with the acquired immunodeficiency syndrome. Submitted for Publication, 1984.
40. P.A. Pizzo, K.J. Robichaud, F.A. Gill, F.G. Witebsky, A.S. Levine, A.B. Deisseroth, D.L. Glaubiger, J.D. Maclowry, I.T. Magrath, D.G. Poplack, and R.M. Simon, Duration of empiric antibiotic therapy in granulocytopenic patients with cancer, Amer.J.Med. 67:194-200 (1979).

IMMUNOMODULATING EFFECTS OF MICROORGANISMS AND THEIR PRODUCTS ON THE IMMUNE RESPONSE MECHANISMS

Herman Friedman

Department of Medical Microbiology and Immunology
University of South Florida College of Medicine
Tampa, Florida

INTRODUCTION

The immune defense system of an individual depends on a complex series of interactions among cells and molecules following exposure of lymphoid cells to specific antigen. Much is now known about the major mechanisms of antibody responses and cell mediated immunity at both the humoral and cellular levels. The magnitude and range of the immune response to a specific antigen are regulated by a wide variety of factors, including soluble mediators derived from various cell types which serve as additional signals to the immune response mechanisms. In this regard, microorganisms and their products, including those derived from Gram-negative and Gram-positive bacteria, are known to exert marked influences on the immune response system of animals and man, both in vivo and in vitro[2,8,11]. Microbial products have been shown to either enhance or suppress the immune response as well as to modify the nature of the response. In addition, many microbial agents, especially viruses, are now known to have the ability to markedly influence the immune response mechanisms, both at the cellular and humoral levels[1,3,4,7,9,10]. In addition, all other microbial classes, including fungi and yeasts, rickettsiae, and single or multiple cellular parasites, are also known to affect immune competence. Besides stimulating specific immune responses to the microorganism itself, antigens derived from many of these microbes are now known to affect in a negative or positive manner a wide range of immune responses.

Polyclonal adjuvantic effects of bacteria and viruses, as well as the immunoderegulation occurring in many microbial infections, are important characteristics of the interaction of microorganisms with a host. In this regard, the effects of a given microbial agent or its products may be on the afferent limb of the immune response arc, the sensitization phase or, in contrast, on the efferent or effector phase. It is often difficult to ascertain which phase if any is involved and frequently both may be influenced by a microbial agent. Moreover, the specific mechanism of action on the immune system may be difficult to ascertain. For example, the sensitization stage or disposition of specific antigen to which an individual is responding may be altered or there may be a direct effect on cells participating in the reaction, i.e., macrophages, T or B lymphocytes, etc. On the affector phase of the humoral immune response, qualitative changes in antibody functional activities, alterations in activation of classic and alternative complement pathways, or changes in the release or action of pharmacological mediators may occur. In reactions of cell mediated immunity, the affector cells, i.e., lymphocytes or macrophages, as well as their products, may be affected by microbial agents.

This review will be limited to a general discussion of the effects of selected bacteria and viruses on the immune response system, especially in regards to predisposing immunodeficiency of the host infected with a microorganism, either a bacterium or virus, and in terms of altered immune competence and dysfunction.

GENERAL EFFECTS OF MICROORGANISM ON THE IMMUNE RESPONSE SYSTEM

The immune response system, especially its interaction with microbes, is being increasingly investigated since it is apparent that immune competence of a normal individual depends upon a complex network of interdependent components. A comprehensive knowledge of the immune system depends upon analyses of each of these components as well as the mechanisms of their interactions. Knowledge of the nature of the immune response provides an essential basis for understanding the mechanism of how a microbe interacts with the immune system. The basic mechanisms controlling different types of immune responses resulting from challenge with a microbe are complex. An imbalance of hemostasis and deregulation of lymphoid cell proliferation and maturation often occurs during infection or exposure of an individual to microbial agents. The lymphoid system is highly dynamic and regulated by an intricate network of interactions among different cells, including lymphoid cells and accessory cells, as well as between cells and soluble mediators, antibodies, antibody-antigen complexes and idiotype-antiidiotype networks.

Lymphoid cells capable of recognizing antigens serve a central role in the immune system and may be divided into two major sublines: a) B-cells (bone marrow derived) i.e., lymphocytes that express antibody molecules on their surface and can be induced to produce and secrete antibodies; and b) T cells, i.e., stem cells "educated" in the thymus to recognize specific antigens in conjunction with cell surface proteins coded for by the major histocompatibility complex.

T cells may be divided into several subsets which carry out different effector cells functions. Some T cells mediate local delayed hypersensitivity reactions, others are cytotoxic and lyse either cells infected with an intracellular microbe or tumor cells. Other regulatory T cells may help or suppress different immune responses affected by other lymphoid cell populations. These T cell populations vary in phenotypic expression of defined surface proteins but the nature of the T cell receptor remains elusive. The B cell population is also heterogeneous and evidence for several functionally separate subsets of B cells has accumulated. B cell subsets are defined by differential responsiveness to a selection of antigens, either directly or by means of T cells. B cells with suppressive activity have been described in a number of systems in the absence of antibody involvement. However, it is evident that antibody can inhibit the generation of effector T cells and exert a feedback control.

Following antigenic challenge, both T and B cells divide and differentiate, resulting in antigen reactive populations of memory cells, and also mature into cells that carry out effector functions, such as antibody secretion or target cell killing. In addition to T and B lymphoid cells, which are responsible for recognizing both self and non-self antigens, certain accessory cells such as macrophages and natural killer cells are now known to play an important role in responding to various antigens including those derived from microbes, interacting with lymphoid cells as well as controlling their function. Among these various cell populations, macrophages and T cells are important in removing invading microorganisms in the presence of antibodies. The function of the system thus depends on continuous developmental stages in the life of different lymphoid cell populations and a highly complex network of interactions among cells and secretory molecules provided by some of the effector and accessory cells regulating the system.

During the normal immune response, the network is finally balanced to permit the induction of different types of immune responses as required, followed by additional responses leaving the host with memory T and B cells. The development of immunological memory occurs rapidly following exposure to a microorganism or other antigens and reflects the ability of the host to respond more rapidly and effectively to a subsequent encounter with the same antigen because more cells, at an advanced level of development, are available to interact specifically with the antigen.

It should be noted that immune balance may be readily perturbed during an infection, potentially leading the host to show altered control of lymphoid cell function. Examples of the presence of persistent virus infection despite immunological responses is well known in infections by viruses such as hepatitis B, herpesviruses, parainfluenza viruses, etc.[1,9]. Similar events may occur with intracellular microbial infections[2,11]. Possible mechanisms enabling the microbe to abrogate the host's immune response involves the localization of the microorganism within sites that are protected from the immune response of the host, but quite often may be due to a direct effect of the microorganism on the immune response, depressing specific or nonspecific reactions. A general discussion of how bacteria and viruses may influence the different pathways of the immune response system is presented below.

EFFECTS OF BACTERIA AND THEIR PRODUCTS ON IMMUNITY

It is widely acknowledged that many bacteria, both Gram-negative or positive, may influence the immune response mechanisms either by directly infecting cells of the immune response system or releasing soluble substances which have immunomodulatory properties. Numerous studies in recent years have been concerned with the adjuvantic activity of bacteria and their products as well as the general or selected immunostimulatory or suppressive properties of such organisms. Considerable work has been concerned with the action of immunomodulatory components of bacteria. A common mechanism so far has not been elucidated and it is probable that different microorganisms affect the immune response system in different ways. However, certain mechanisms of action appear to be common in regards to immunostimulation. Many bacteria and their antigens act directly on cells involved in the immune response system. They also may modify the configuration and presentation of antigens, alter the metabolism of antigens by lymphoid cells and, when acting directly on the response system, may interact directly with cells resulting in activation of macrophages, B cells or T cells. Bacteria and their products may affect the immune response by specifically acting on certain cell membrane enzymes causing their activation or inhibition.

In terms of immune suppression, it is quite apparent that most pathogenic bacteria, as well as opportunistic microorganisms in general, not only must first establish themselves within a host, but must also avoid destruction by the immune response system. Various interactions of bacteria with the host defense system are therefore central to the nature of bacterial virulence. A non-immune host depends upon non-specific defenses such as complement, phagocytosis and nutrient limitation.

Even when specific protective immunity is present, it often functions merely by refining nonspecific mechanisms. It is apparent that defenses against bacterial infections include not only nonspecific humoral defenses based on phagocytosis, complement and other cellular and soluble humoral factors, but also on specific immunity. A brief review of some of the components associated with microorganisms which are now known to be involved in the resistance of a microorganisms against the host defense system is discussed below.

Gram-positive bacteria, including cocci, have long been known to have mechanisms whereby they can elude the host defense system. Among the Gram-positive organisms the staphylococci and streptococci have been studied in some detail in terms of immunomodulatory factors. As indicated in Table 1, staphylococcal extracellular or surface components such as capsules or clumping factors, protein A and protein B, as well as many extracellular enzymes including enzymes specific for host serum proteins, blood cell membranes, leukocytes, etc., may influence the immune response in a variety of ways. More recently, it has been shown that the cell wall components of cocci, including peptidogylcan and lipotechoic acids, are strongly immunomodulatory. The host responds to these factors by formation of antibody and specifically-sensitized T lymphocytes. Nevertheless, rapid growth of these bacteria in a susceptible host often results in the release of toxins and cellular components which may depress in a specific or nonspecific manner the host immune system.

Gram negative bacilli, in particular, have been studied in great depth in terms of immunomodulatory activities (Table 1). It is now widely acknowledged that Gram-negative bacilli influence in both a negative as well as positive manner, nonspecific as well as specific host defenses[2,11]. Most of these activities have been associated with the lipopolysaccharide (LPS) structure of the cell walls of these bacteria. Such LPS may contribute to resistance of most Gram-negative bacteria to complement associated lysis[8]. This may be due to superficial branched chain sugar residues of LPS, which may interfere with access of complement to target antigens on the cell envelope. The presence of LPS may also be involved in resistance of some organisms to natural killing by phagocytes. LPS has been studied in much detail immunochemically and is known to be the structural component of cell walls of all Gram-negative bacteria. LPS may serve as a powerful adjuvant for antibody formation in vivo as well as in vitro. It may also abrogate immunologic tolerance and convert a tolerogenic dose of an antigen into an immunogenic one. LPS may also induce nonspecific differentiation of B cells into antibody forming cells, i.e., polyclonal activation. It also may stimulate lymphocytes to produce soluble mediators, as well as macrophages, stimulating their differentiation and inducing them to produce a wide variety of soluble immunostimulatory molecules.

Table 1. Bacterial Factors Affecting Immune Responses

BACTERIA	FACTOR
Gram-Positive Cocci	
Staphylococci	Capsule, clumping factor, Protein A and B, teichoic acid
Streptococci	Lipoteichoic acid, membrane enzymes, pyrogenic exotoxin, peptidoglycans
Pneumococci	Capsule, cell wall
Gram-Negative Cocci	
Neisseria	Cell walls, cord factor, exotoxins
Other Bacteria	
Mycobacteria Cornebacteria	Cell walls, cord factor, peptidoglycans, MDP
Gram Negative Bacilli	
Enterobacteriaceae, Vibrios, Pertussis	Lipopolysaccharide, cell wall components, exotoxins

In vitro treatment of macrophages with LPS activates these cells to produce essentially all of their currently recognized products, including lymphocyte activating factors, i.e., interleukin 1, which acts on T lymphocytes, interferons, colony stimulating factors, prostaglandins, and cellular metabolism factors, as well as other factors.

Although the effects of LPS on B lymphocytes and macrophages are now well established, until recently it was not generally appreciated that LPS may act on T lymphocytes as well. It is now known that the lipid A moiety of LPS enhances the differentiation of thymus populations in vitro. In terms of LPS induced adjuvanticity, it has been found that in vitro stimulation may be mediated by effects on T lymphocytes and macrophages. This does not necessarily depend on direct effects on these cells. LPS stimulation of macrophages may result in release of factors such as lymphocyte activating factor, and may also result in stimulation of T cells to produce immunostimulatory proteins such as T cell replacing factor or interleukin 2.

Mycobacteria have been studied in great detail in terms of their effects on immune responses (Table 1). Mycobacterial antigens in particular have been incorporated into oils and such preparations have been considered among the most potent stimulants in increasing antibody levels and also potentiating production of delayed hypersenstivity reactions. Recently the chemical structure responsible for the adjuvantic activity of mycobacteria has been elucidated and is similar to the active material involved in the adjuvantic activity and immunoregulatory properties of many other microorganisms. The peptidoglycan lipid material associated with the wax D of these bacteria was utilized to obtain a water soluble nitrogenous material with adjuvantic activity[6]. This nitrogen-containing fraction was characterized by Lederer and associates in France and by Kotani and collaborators in Japan, as the minimal adjuvantic component of bacterial cell walls. This material has been identified as N-acetylmuramyl-L-alanyl-D-isoglutamine (MDP) and can replace mycobacteria in oil adjuvants and has as its primary target macrophages which release monokines which, in turn, activate B and T cells[6].

It is widely recognized that other bacteria have marked immunoregulatory activities. For example, soluble Bordetella pertussis extracts affect both specific and nonspecific immune responses. Soluble extracts are rich in both endotoxins and exotoxins. The exotoxins in particular preferentially augment IgG as well as IgE antibody formation. This may result from direct stimulatory effects on T and B cells. Macrophage activating activity has also been found in pertussis extracts. Many immunostimulatory properties of pertussis appear to reside in the same components responsible for pharmacological effects.

INFLUENCE OF VIRUSES ON IMMUNITY

It is widely acknowledged that many viruses may affect the immune responses either in a negative or positive manner[1,3,4,7,9,10]. Many viral infections suppress one or more components of the host defense mechanism. Which components are impaired and to what extent they are impaired, depends on the many variables among which are virus type and strain. The mechanisms, however, which cause such immunosuppression are still poorly defined and probably are highly diverse. Nevertheless, studies with many different viral infectious agents indicate that some generalizations are possible. In most, if not all instances, some insights into mechanisms have shown that immunologic impairment is due to functional alterations of immunocompetent cells (Tables 2-4). These, in turn, may be caused by direct interactions of a virus with lymphoid cells and less frequently by substances produced by other cells as a consequence of viral infection.

Many viruses appear to be endowed with direct immunosuppressive properties. However, different cells may be affected by different viruses. Numerous alterations of immunocompetent cell function have been observed in the course of different viral infections. Such functional alterations do not necessarily presuppose extensive damage of lymphoid tissue. In fact, hyperplastic changes may occur but as a rule, substantially few, if any, histological alterations of lymphoid tissue become evident in viral infection. Nevertheless, in some viral infection, lymphatic tissues show lesions usually limited in scope, which may resemble the cytopathic effects characteristic of the infecting virus in vitro. For instance, during measles infections, typical giant cells may develop in various lymphoid organs beginning at the very early stages of infection. Furthermore, in general, viral infection such as dengue hemorrhagic fever, results in various degrees of cellular depletion which affect specific and distinct areas of the lymphoid tissue.

Table 2. Viruses Known to Replicate in Immunocompetent Cells

VIRUS	CELL TYPES
Poliomyelitis	Mo; L*
Coxsackie B	L+
Echo	Mo; L*
Influenza	Mo; LT (abortive infection)
Parainfluenza	Mo; LT; LB
Measles	Mo; LT*; LB
Mumps	L+
Rubella	Mo; LT
Yellow fever	Mo; LT
Dengue	Mo; LB; LT*
Lymphocytic choriomeningitis	Mo
Adenovirus	L
Herpes simplex	Mo; Lt*; LB*
Varicella zoster	Mo
Cytomegalovirus	Mo; LB
Epstein-Barr	LB
Vaccinia	Mo L*

Mo = macrophages; L = lymphocytes not characterized; LB = B lymphocytes; LT = T lymphocytes; * = viral replication is possible or is substantially potentiated, if cells have been specifically or unspecifically stimulated).

The structural integrity of lymphoid tissue does not prevent immunocompetent cells from exhibiting profound manifestations of functional deficiency. A typical example is the reduced in vitro blastogenic reponses of lymphocytes to specific antigens, mitogens, or alloantigens in many viral infections which are readily reproduced in experimentally infected animals. Among the various other modifications of immunocompetent cell behavior are those of lymphoid cell migration, both in vivo and in vitro. Modifications in lymphocyte traffic are well documented and have contributed to cell surface changes which subsequently reduce the ability of affected cells to interact with either endothelial cells of vessels or other reticuloendothelial cells. Altered cell traffic patterns may account for the fluctuations of peripheral blood leukocyte counts which occur in many viral diseases and which remain unexplained. It is widely recognized that lymphopenia occurs in various virus infections such as those induced by measles, rubella, varicella, poliomyelitis and influenza, as well as those caused by coxsackievirus, adenovirus and arbovirus infections. Transient lymphopenia may be present in early stages of viral infections and may become pronounced, affecting all or only selected cell populations.

It seems likely that the major mechanisms whereby immunocompetent cell alterations occur in virus infections may be associated with either direct activity of the virus or an indirect one mediated by soluble factors (Table 4). Direct action of the virus may occur, expecially in acute phases of infection where virus sometimes is isolated from peripheral blood leukocytes. Many viruses are capable of replicating within immunocompetent cells (Table 2). Various studies have permitted recognition of the cellular types and specific subtypes of lymphoid cells susceptible to virus infections. Experiments in vitro in which various immunocompetent cell classes have been infected have proven fruitful in providing new information concerning virus-cell interactions and the possible regulatory factors involved.

It has been established that the outcome of the interaction between a virus and an immunocompetent cell markedly depends upon the metabolic state of the target cell itself, possible more so than with the virus type (1). Thus, macrophages, often restricted for many viruses, may undergo changes in susceptibility to virus infection once specifically activated through signals emitted by lymphocytes. In turn, the latter cells, if placed in contact with a virus while in the quiescent state, very often result in abortive infection followed by incomplete synthesis of virus

immunocompetent cells have been observed repeatedly. Soluble substances toxic for lymphocytes have been found in various patients in the acute phase of different viral infections (Table 3). Furthermore, it has been found that serum factors nonspecific-

Table 3. Parameters of Immunological Responsiveness Suppressed During Viral Infections

IMMUNE PARAMETER	VIRUS
Ig levels in serum	Congenital rubella
Antibody response	Many
Antibody-dependent hypersensitivity	Junin
Circulating autoantibody	Reovirus, selected retroviruses
Spontanteous autoimmune lesions	Lactic dehydrogenase virus
Cell-mediated hypersensitivity	Many
Contact sensitivity	Polio, Coxsackie B, mumps, measles, Epstein-Barr
T-cell-mediated cytotoxicity	Selected retroviruses
Skin allograft rejection	Cytomegalovirus (murine), Marek
Graft-versus-host induction	Dengue
Immunological maturation	Lymphocytic choriomeningitis
Tolerance induction	Venzuelan equine encephalitis, lymphocytic choriomeningitis
Lymphocyte and antigen trapping by spleen	Lactic dehydrogenase virus
Resistance to superinfection	Cytomegalovirus, influenza, measles, parainfluenza
Resistance to tumor induction or growth	Cytomegalovirus (murine), lactic dehydrogenase virus

ally inhibiting cell mediated responses may occur in patients with infectious mononucleosis or hepatitis. Although such factors appear not to be viral components, their exact chemical nature and role have yet to be defined. In addition, tissues outside the immune system may release substances during virus infection which affect the immune responsiveness. This is exemplified by fibroblast interferon which is endowed with distinct immunomodulatory properties. Similarly, the gamma-interferon released by certain activated lymphocytes also has immunoregulatory properties that may be induced by virus infections. It should be noted, finally, that some of the pathogenesis associated with virus-induced immunomodulation may be due to autoimmune "phenomena" in which viral antigens are expressed on lymphoid cell surfaces. These antigens may then be recognized by other immunocompetent host cells, which then react against lymphoid cells bearing the virus antigen. Such cells, even though functionally normal despite their virus infection or expression of viral antigen, are then destroyed or inactivated, resulting in net loss of immunocompetent cells and/or immunologic determination.

Table 4. Some Stratagems, Other than Immunosuppression and Immunocompetent Cell Invasion, that Allow Viruses to Elude Host Immune Defenses

Integration in unexpressed form into host cell DNA	Papovaviruses, retroviruses
Intracytoplasmic latency with occasional reactivation concomitant with declines in host resistance	Herpes simplex, varicella - zoster
Direct cell-to-cell spread	Herpes simplex, cytomegalovirus
Budding on intracellular membranes	Coronaviruses
Antigenic drift	Influenza, visna
Deletion of virion envelope genes	Defective retroviruses
Propagation as naked genomes	Putative viroids (rheumatoid arthritis)
Incorporation of host antigens in virion envelope	Retroviruses
Lack of stimulation of immune responses	Unconventional viruses (spongiform encephalopathies)
Partial tolerance	Lymphocytic choriomeningitis, rubella
Induction of non-neutralizing antibodies that hinder neutralization or facilitate viropexis	Lactic dehydrogenase virus, dengue, reoviruses
Production of excess soluble antigens that compete with virions for immune effectors	Hepatitis B
Depression of response to interferon induction	Cytomegalovirus, lymphocytic choriomeningitis, selected retroviruses
Low sensitivity to interferon	Adenoviruses
Induction of anticomplementary factors	Junin virus
Invasion of body districts in which immune effectors are weak (skin, exocrine glands, kidney, CNS)	Papilloma, mumps, Creutzfeld-Jakob, KB, measles

DISCUSSION AND CONCLUSIONS

It has now become widely appreciated that the interaction of microorganism and a host is a two-way reaction in that the host attempts to respond to the microbe by preventing attachment, colonization and eventually infection and, in turn, the microbe attempts to subvert the defense mechanism of the host in order to establish a foothold. Over the millions of years of natural selection of a host and its parasites, a symbiotic relationship has developed in which most microorganisms, after establishment within a certain species, do not cause harmful effects. In turn, much of the responsiveness of the host to microorganisms may actually be of benefit to the host in that the immune system develops, matures, and becomes competent only after constant exposure to normal flora from birth onwards. In terms of possible detrimental effects, it is now apparent that microorganisms interact with nonspecific host defenses by developing methods to avoid complement and antibody-associated lysis and utilizing nutritional and environmental factors from the host for their own benefit. The host, in turn, may resist invasion by a microorganism, even after colonization has occurred, by mobilization of bone marrow-derived cells necessary for nonspecific immune defenses as well as by inflammatory and chemotactic reactions to the invading microorganism, opsonization of the microbe by humoral antibody and complement, phagocytosis, and finally, intracellular killing of those organisms which penetrate into the host proper and intracellular millieu. As a consequence, many microorganisms, especially pathogenic ones, have evolved "virulence" factors and they are often capable of overcoming some or all portions of the host defense system. These include genetically and phenotypically programmed microbial factors such as capsules, cell wall components and extracellular products which may either prevent the microorganism from being recognized and opsonized by the host and/or actively subvert the immune response system.

Many factors associated with different pathogenic microorganisms as well as opportunistic pathogens and normal flora are now known to be immunomodulatory. It is now widely recognized that relatively small amounts of many bacterial products, as well as virus components, may serve as potent stimulators of specific components of the host defense responses, including phagocytic reactions, B and T lymphocyte activities and macrophage function. It is important to note, however, that there are relatively large amounts of the same components which have also been found in many cases to be immunosuppressive and to block various host immune defenses. Thus, there is a crucial balance between the responses of the host to a relatively small quantity of microorganisms or their products vs. the inability of the host and its defense mechanism to be activated or respond in a productive manner to larger amounts of the same products. A further understanding of the complex interactions between microorganisms, including bacteria and viruses, with the host defense system is necessary to develop a more rational basis for successful treatment of infectious agents, especially those which are associated with immune deficiency. With the advent of many immunorestorative substances and development of new knowledge in the area of immunopharmacology and immunobiology in general, a better understanding of basic interactions between microbes and the host immune system is evolving so that the appropriate strategy may be developed to tip the balance of the host-parasite relationship in favor of the host during infectious diseases.

REFERENCES

1. Bendinelli, M., Mechanisms and significance of immuno-depression in viral diseases. Clin. Immunol. Newsletter 2:75-80, (1981).
2. Friedman, H., Klein, T. W. and Szentivanyi, A., Immunomodulation by Bacteria and their products, Plenum Press, NY, (1981).
3. Friedman, H. and Specter, S., Virus induced immunomodulation, in Advances in Immunopharmacology, J. Hadden, L. Chedid, P. Muller and F. Spreafico, eds., Pergammon Press, NY, pp. 91-100, (1981).
4. Friedman, H., Specter, S., Farber, P. and Ceglowski, W., Interactions of viruses with lymphoid cells, in, Cell Biology and Immunology of Leukocyte Function, Academic Press, NY, pp. 783-802, (1979)
5. Kotani, S., Watanabi, Y., Kioshita, F., Shimono, T., Morisaki, I., Shiba, T., Kusumoto, S., Tarumi, Y. and Ikenaka, K., Immunoadjuvant activities of synthetic N-acetylmuramylpeptides or amino acids. Bikin J. 18:105, (1975).
6. Lederer, E., Immunomodulation by muramyl peptides, recent developments, Clin. Immun. Newsletter 3:83, (1982).
7. Proffitt, M.R., Virus-lymphocyte interactions: Implications for disease, Elsevier/North-Holland, NY, (1979).
8. Schwab, J. H., Acute and chronic inflammation induced by bacterial cell wall structures, in Microbiology, D. Schlesinger, ed., Amer. Soc. Microbiol., Wash., DC, pp. 209-214, (1979).
9. Specter, S. and Friedman, H., Viruses and the immune response, Pharmac. Ther. A , 2:595-622, (1978).
10. Woodruff, J. F. and Woodruff, J. J., T lymphocyte interaction with virus and virus-infected tissues, Prog. Med. Virol. 19:120-160, (1975).
11. Yamamura, Y., Kotani, S., Azuma, T., Koda, A. and Shiba, T., Immunomodulation by Microbial Products and Related Synthetic Components, Excerpta Medica, Amsterdam, (1982).

THE DIAGNOSIS AND DEFINITION OF THE ACQUIRED IMMUNODEFICIENCY SYNDROME*

James A. Hoxie

Department of Medicine, University of Pennsylvania School of Medicine, Philadelphia, PA

INTRODUCTION

Since June 1981, the acquired immunodeficiency syndrome (AIDS) has been reported in over 10,000 individuals in the United States and in over 500 individuals from other countries. Epidemiologic evidence has suggested that a new transmissible agent is, at least in part, responsible. The Center for Disease Control (CDC) has defined this syndrome as the occurrence of opportunistic infections or Kaposi's sarcoma in previously healthy individuals less than 60 years of age with no other underlying medical condition or therapy associated with immunodeficiency. This surveillance definition has been easily applied by clinicians from a variety of backgrounds and has been useful in monitoring the evolution of this epidemic at the national level. It has helped to define major risk groups in the population with approximately 95% of cases continuing to be restricted to homosexual or bisexual males, intravenous drug users, hemophiliacs. However, the full extent of this problem is undoubtedly underestimated by this definition. In areas where AIDS is endemic, a syndrome which includes unexplained persisting generalized lymphadenopathy or a chronic wasting syndrome has also been increasingly recognized, principally in the major risk groups noted[1-3]. One prospective study has demonstrated that as high as 15% of such individuals will either develop AIDS as defined by the CDC or lymphomas, and raises the concern that a poorly defined AIDS-related disorder currently exists affecting a larger population[1]. The scope of this problem is further complicated by case reports suggesting possible carrier states in asymptomatic individuals capable of transmitting the disease[4-6] and by the recognition of a related syndrome in infants born principally to mothers who are Haitian or intravenous drug users[7,8].

*Editor's note: The Chapter represents the state of knowledge of AIDS in 1983. A brief addendum follows the text.

Delineating the full spectrum of AIDS will ultimately require a broadened definition which relates complex immunologic, virologic, and clinical abnormalities to the natural history of AIDS and related disorders. Common to all affected individuals with the fully developed syndrome has been a severe and thus far irreversible depression of the host immune system. The complexity of these abnormalities likely relates to the combined effects of the etiologic agent in AIDS and the immunosuppressive effects of secondary de novo or reactivated viral infections. This report will review the characteristic immunologic abnormalities seen in CDC-defined AIDS and summarize the clinical and laboratory characteristics of these other AIDS-related disorders.

Early descriptions of AIDS occurring with opportunistic infections recognized profound deficits in cellular immunity[9-12]. Patients were anergic to a variety of recall antigens and in vitro their T cells demonstrated hyporesponsiveness to mitogens soluble antigens, and to alloantigens. Lymphopenia was seen frequently and analysis with monoclonal antibodies to T cell subsets demonstrated a marked reduction in the relative and absolute number of helper/inducer T cells reactive with the antibodies OKT4 or Leu-3a. In the setting of normal absolute numbers and a relative increased percentage of suppressor/cytotoxic T cells reactive with OKT8 or Leu-2a, severe reductions in the "helper to suppressor cell ratio" or T4/T8 ratio were seen. Normally, about 2.0, T4/T8 ratios less than 0.1 were often present in patients whose primary disease manifestation was opportunistic infection. Less severe but significant reductions were seen in patients presenting with Kaposi's sarcoma alone without opportunistic infections (13). Limited reports of functional studies have indicated that T4 cells are not only reduced in number but are qualitatively defective in their ability to provide help to B cells in immunoglobulin production. T8 cells, on the other hand, were shown to have normal suppressor function in this assay[14]. Less severe but significant alterations in T lymphocyte subsets and proliferative capacity have been reported in homosexual men from endemic areas with a syndrome characterized by chronic (>3-6 months), unexplained generalized lymphadenopathy[2,13,15].

Others have noted mild but significant reductions in the helper/suppressor ratio in asymptomatic homosexual men from endemic[16,17] but not nonendemic areas[18]. Although the progressive decline in T4/T8 ratios seen in these groups suggest a related disorder differing only in severity, the nonspecificity of this alteration, which can be seen particularly in viral infections common among homosexual men, has complicated the interpretation of these results. Fahey has drawn attention to the absolute numbers of T cell subsets rather than percentages and has suggested that a low helper/suppressor cell ratio in asymptomatic homosexual men is usually due to an increased number of suppressor cells (T suppressor cell augmentation) rather than a low number of T helper cells (T helper cell depletion) seen in AIDS patients[19,20]. Prospective studies in progress at several centers will help to determine among patients with the generalized lymphadenopathy syndrome if a low ratio due to T helper cell depletion differs prognostically from a low ratio due to T suppressor cell augmentation.

Numerous other T cell abnormalities have been demonstrated in AIDS. A defect in the ability of T cells from AIDS patients to kill skin fibroblasts infected with cytomegalovirus was described by Rook demonstrating an impaired cytotoxic effector mechanism[21]. Interestingly, this defect was corrected in vitro by the use of the lymphokine interleukin-2 (IL-2) and has provided a rationale for clinical trials using IL-2 as therapy in AIDS. T lymphocytes have also shown an inability to produce and respond to interferons. In addition, several serum suppressor factors are being investigated which may potentiate these defects including antilymphocyte antibodies[22,23], monocyte-derived suppressor factors[24], and a low molecular weight factor termed CY-AIDS detected in four AIDS patients which biochemically bears some similarity to cyclosporins which are well recognized as potent immunosuppressive compounds[25]. Cellular interactions may also participate in the impaired T cell function. Activated circulating radiosensitive suppressor cells which inhibited T proliferative responses to concanavalin A have been demonstrated by Hersh[26]. Indeed, the major circulating T cells in AIDS characterized by opportunistic infections have acquired antigens expressed on activated, but not resting T cells, suggesting a role for these cells in disease pathogenesis[27].

In addition to T cell abnormalities, a wide variety of humoral immune defects are also present in AIDS. Patients characteristically show polyclonal hypergammaglobulinemia with more than 90% having an elevation in at least one immunoglobulin type[16]. Paradoxically these individuals exhibit depressed antibody responses to recall and de novo antigens. In vitro, B cells have been demonstrated to spontaneously secrete immunoglobulin while at the same time show depressed antibody production to the T cell-dependent B cell activator, pokeweed mitogen, and to the T cell-independent mitogen, Staphylococcus aureus Cowan Strain I. As suggested by Lane and Fauci, these in vivo and in vitro abnormalities are consistent with a preactivation of circulating B cells which spontaneously secrete immunoglobulin and become resistant to further stimulation[14]. The mechanism for this is unknown but may relate to the reactivation of the Epstein-Barr virus, well known to be a potent B cell stimulator. Serologic evidence for past or reactivated EBV infection is universally present in AIDS patients. Moreover, a role for this virus in the pathogenesis but not necessarily the cause of AIDS, is suggested by marked elevations in anti-EBV titers in many of these individuals and in the detection of EBV genome in B cell lymphomas arising from AIDS patients[28]. An alternate explanation for the excessive B cell stimulation in AIDS may relate to the recent observation that cytomegalovirus can activate B cell immunoglobulin production independent of T cells[29]. Serological evidence of past CMV infection with this virus is present in virtually all homosexual men with AIDS and in the majority can be cultured from either blood, urine, saliva, or semen[30].

Several serological abnormalities have been described which may in combination with previously mentioned cellular abnormalities allow a better laboratory definition and detection of AIDS. Several reports have demonstrated an unusual form of alpha-interferon which is acid-labile in 68-100% of patients with AIDS[31-33]. Of interest was its detection in two hemophiliacs, three and ten months before the clinical diagnosis of AIDS[32]. Similar observations were reported by Blumovici-Klein in which five homosexual men developed AIDS 2-17 months after elevated levels of acid-labile interferon were detected[31]. Zolla-Pazner has, in addition, demonstrated marked elevations in serum beta-2 microglobulin levels in all patients with either AIDS or suspected of having AIDS because of persisting unexplained lymphadenopathy, oral thrush, or weight loss[34]. Interestingly, among a group of 40 asymptomatic homosexual men followed prospectively, seven were found to have elevated beta-2 microglobulin levels and of these, six subsequently developed either AIDS or suspected AIDS as defined above. The other 33 individuals remained well.

Increases in serum alpha-1 thymosin levels have been described in AIDS as another potential disease marker. Produced by the thymus, this hormone promotes the maturation of helper T cells and has been postulated by Goldstein to increase as the result of end organ failure from the progresive reduction in T cell number or function[35]. Over 85% of patients with AIDS were found to have elevated levels of this hormone and 30-40% of immunologically abnormal homosexual men in Houston and Denmark also had increased levels[36].

The ability to diagnose AIDS would, of course, be greatly facilitated if the etiologic agent or agents could be identified. (Refer to Addendum.) Recent reports have suggested a role for the human T cell leukemia virus (HTLV) in the pathogenesis of AIDS and have drawn considerable attention in developing assays for HTLV infection[37-39]. This type C retrovirus has been well associated with a distinct form of T cell leukemia endemic in southwestern Japan and in the West Indies and has had sporadic association with other T cell malignancies in the United States. The rationale for implicating HTLV in AIDS is based on 1) the recognized ability of HTLV to be transmitted horizontally among close family contacts, 2) its predeliction for transforming and presumably infecting helper T cells which are, as mentioned, severly deficient in AIDS, and 3) the well documented association of other animal leukemia retroviruses with immunodeficiency syndromes. As reported by Essex, antibodies to HTLV membrane-associated antigens have been detected in 25-33% of homosexual men with AIDS, compared to less than 1% of asymptomatic homosexual men or heterosexual controls[37]. Similar results have been reported by hemophiliacs where 5-19% of individuals were positive using this assay[40]. Infectious HTLV virus has been demonstrated in lymphocytes from some homosexual and hemophiliac patients with AIDS, although this has been found in the minority[39,41]. While these studies demonstrate an association of HTLV with AIDS, it remains unclear if this virus or a related virus is the cause or simply a secondary opportunistic infection in an already immunodeficient host.

It is important to recognize that none of the laboratory tests already mentioned have the sensitivity or specificity to be used as a diagnostic test for AIDS. Lymphocyte subsets are altered by numerous infections including cytomegalovirus, Epstein-Barr virus, hepatitis B, rhinovirus, influenza and toxoplasmosis. Acid-labile interferon is also elevated in some autoimmune disorders and beta-2 microglobulin increases are seen in B cell malignancies, systemic lupus erythematosis and sarcoidosis. Alpha-1 thymosin elevations are seen in multiple sclerosis and some neoplasms, and positive HTLV serologies can be demonstrated in as high as 15% of population in HTLV endemic areas, such as southwestern Japan or the Carribean basin. In addition, the use of these tests in non-AIDS control groups with viral and protozoan infections must be assessed to completely evaluate their specificity and utility as markers in AIDS. However, while no one test may be specific for AIDS, the possibility exists that in the absence of a detectable etiologic agent several tests may be used in combination. Efforts are in progess at several centers to generate immunologic and serologic profiles of "surrogate markers" for this syndrome.

A more specific panel of laboratory tests for AIDS is crucial to a complete delineation of the full extent of this problem in groups not included in the current CDC definition. One group of particular concern is homosexual men with sustained (more than 3 months) generalized (more than 2 extra inguinal sites) lymphadenopathy[1-3]. Such individuals experience a variety of symptoms including fatigue, weight loss, night sweats, myalgias, headache, and diarrhea. Lymph nodes which may vary in size from 1 cm to 5 cm typically wax and wane over time and are associated with splenomegaly on physical exam in 20-30% of all patients. Interestingly, one-fourth of patients in one series gave a history of an acute viral illness preceding the onset of the syndrome[1]. Lymph node biopsies typically show a nonspecific pattern of florid reactive hyperplasia, or less commonly, a pattern of follicular involution with depletion of germinal centers[1,42,43]. This latter histology, although seen in the minority, typically occurs in the setting of severe immunodeficiency and frequently precedes a diagnosis of AIDS[1]. Laboratory abnormalities are nonspecific and include hypergammaglobulinemia, positive antinuclear antibodies, anemia or leukopenia in less than 10%, and a low T4/T8 ratio which unlike most viral illnesses is typically due to a reduction in T4 cell number with or without an increase in T8 cells[1,2,44].

The true incidence of this syndrome, its natural history, and relationship to AIDS currently are unknown. The number of affected individuals in all likelihood greatly exceed those diagnosed as having AIDS. Prospective studies of patients in several centers have shown as many as 2-15% of these individuals develop AIDS during a two year period[1,3,44]. Of note, although most patients have remained clinically unchanged with abnormal but stable laboratory tests, resolution of the clinical syndrome or associated immune abnormalities has been uncommon. the use of laboratory tests such as those previously described, may provide a means to determine which individuals within this heterogeneous group are at greatest risk of ultimately developing AIDS. Carefully controlled prospective studies will be needed to answer these important questions. One group of patients presenting clinically with a wasting syndrome appears to be at particular risk for developing AIDS. AS described by Mathur, these patients have marked weight loss, diarrhea, fever for more than 6 months, and persisting thrush with or without adenopathy[45]. Thirty-three of 43 (77%) such patients were seen to develop AIDS in 1-20 months (median 4) suggesting that this entity may be a true AIDS prodrome..

Several recent reports have indicated that patients with either AIDS or persisting generalized lymphadenopathy are at increased risk for developing non-Hodgkin's lymphomas. Since 1981 over 50 cases of lymphoma have occurred in homosexual men with these syndromes in New York City, Los Angeles, and San Francisco alone[1,28,46-48]. An increased frequency of extramedullary presentation with central nervous system involvement and infectious complications during therapy has been noted along with a poor response to conventional chemotherapy. The malignancies are typically of B cell origin and are aggressive histologically including Burkitt's, diffuse histiocytic and immunoblastic sarcoma subtypes. Epstein-Barr viral antigens and DNA have been found in the malignant tissue of some lymphomas suggesting its role in the pathogenesis of this neoplasm[28]. This process may be analogous to EBV-associated lymphomas arising in other immunosuppressed hosts such as renal transplant patients[49] or in the primary X-linked immunodeficiency syndrome[50]. The occurrence of this problem both in patients with AIDS and in the lymphadenopathy syndrome again underscores the urgent need of delineating the critical immunologic abnormalities common to both disorders and requisite for the evolution of this syndrome.

Additional evidence suggests that the full spectrum of AIDS may include an asymptomatic carrier state in which individuals in risk groups may be clinically well but capable of transmitting the disease to other unaffected individuals[4-6,51]. One well publicized example is of an infant in San Francisco who received multiple blood and platelet transfusions at birth and six months later subsequently developed severe immunodeficiency eventually complicated by candida dermatitis, thrush, disseminated Mycobacterium avium-intracellulare, Pneumocystis carinii pneumonia, and death at age 2. One donor, although well at the time of phlebotomy, was a homosexual man who seven months later developed AIDS complicated by cytomegalovirus pneumonia, lymphadenopathy, and P. carinii pneumonia. Five of these contacts occurred when the index individual was asymptomatic and two occurred while he had lymphadenopathy, again suggesting but not proving a preclinical carrier state[51]. One recent report from the CDC evaluated 18 cases of AIDS which developed following multiple blood transfusions[5]. In the seven cases where all donors have been evaluated, at least one donor could be identified who either was in a high risk group for AIDS or had a low T helper/suppressor cell ratio. In five of these cases, at risk donors were homosexual men with multiple sexual partners and a low ratio.

The previously described case of the infant developing a syndrome similar if not identical to AIDS following blood transfusions also indicated that transmission to neonates was possible. Subsequently, over 40 cases of a pediatric AIDS-like syndrome have been reported further broadening the scope of this epidemic[7,8,52,53]. These individuals typically present with evidence of immunological dysfunction at a mean of six months of age, clinically manifested as failure to thrive, recurrent bacterial and viral infections, thrush, lymphadenopathy, splenomegaly, parotitis, P. carinii pneumonia, and frequently an idiopathic interstitial pneumonia. As in adults with AIDS, low helper/suppressor cell ratios, hypergammaglobulinemia, and profound T cell hyporesponsiveness are typical. The majority of these reported cases have been born to mothers who were intravenous drug users or Haitian, many of whom had either CDC-defined AIDS or a generalized lymphadenopathy with some evidence of immune dysfunction. these cases have suggested that AIDS may be transmitted not only by intimate sexual contact or parenterally by needles or blood products, but also in utero or perinatally. One report described an apparent familial clustering of AIDS and related disorders[54]. The mother, an intravenous drug user, died with P. carinii pneumonia and a lymphoma; the father had generalized lymphadenopathy and anergy; a one year old son had genralized lymphadenopathy, splenomegaly, and chronic pulmonary infiltrates, and his four year old sister had lymphadenopathy, splenomegaly, pumonary infiltrates, and anergy. All had markedly low helper/suppressor cell ratios less than 0.4 and were hypergammaglobulinemic. Clearly, while in utero transmission remains possible, important questions remain concerning both the course of these apparent AIDS-related disorders and modes of transmission within such families.

Such epidemiological evidence has strongly suggested that a new syndrome of acquired immune deficiency exists in children whose mothers either have AIDS or are in risk groups. However, these cases must be distinguished from inherited immune disorders such as Nezelof's syndrome which may occur with combined defects in cellular and humoral immunity. As described by Rubenstein, pediatric AIDS appears to be distinct ffom congenital immunodeficiencies and can be linked to the epidemic in adults because 1) it has been reported in geographical areas where AIDS is endemic, 2) impaired cell mediated immunity with hypergammaglobulinemia is uncommon among congenital immune disorders, and 3) in nearly all cases, similar immune abnormalities or AIDS have been present in mothers suggesting a transmitted rather than congenital disorder[53]. Moreover, in one recent report, lymphadenopathic Kaposi's sarcoma occurred in two pediatric AIDS cases born to Haitian parents[52]. However, as in adults with AIDS, many questions remain as to the criteria needed for diagnosing this syndrome and related disorders as they are manifested in children.

This brief review of laboratory abnormalities and clinical features associated with the AIDS-related disorders has emphasized several points. Although AIDS is presently diagnosed by appropriate infections or Kaposi's sarcoma occurring in a previously normal host, the abnormalities which predispose to this are likely initiated well before this diagnosis is established. The detection of carrier states and preclinical forms of AIDS are crucial tasks facing researchers in this field. In addition to the need to define earlier forms of this syndrome, of equal importance is the delineation of the natural history of these entities in children an adults. How many exposed individuals will become infectious? How many individuals with the generalized lymphadenopathy syndrome will progress to AIDS? While no one laboratory test currently offers a specific diagnosis for AIDS or for exposed individuals destined to develop it, combinations of these tests may hold some promise for both prognostic purposes as well as in elucidating the pathogenesis of this disease. Such a broad approach must suffice pending a more direct means of identifying the presumed etiologic agent. In addition, it is likely that in time more indolent forms of this syndrome will be identified. Even the natural history of CDC-defined AIDS remains to be fully delineated. Some individuals presenting with AIDS, complicated by Kaposi's sarcoma alone, may not pursue the aggressive and rapidly fatal course typical for those presenting with opportunistic infections. The answers to these and other questions will require the continuing combined efforts of basic scientific researchers and clinicians and ultimately the time to completely evaluate the complex laboratory abnormalities and the full clinical spectrum of AIDS.

ADDENDUM

Since this symposium on infections in the compromised host was held in November, 1983, dramatic progess has been made in identifying the probable etiologic agent in AIDS. Reports from several laboratories have described the isolation of a new group of retroviruses from patients with AIDS. These have been termed human T-lymphotropic virus type-III (HTLV-III)[55-57], lymphadenopathy-associated virus (LAV)[58-59], and AIDS-associated retrovirus (ARV)[60]. Several of these isolates have been molecularly cloned, and both restriction endonuclease mapping and sequence analysis has shown them to be closely related to each other while at the same time distinct from other known retroviruses[61-66]. A distant relationship to the previously mentioned transforming viruses now termed HTLV-1 has been proposed[61-66] but this remains controversial[62,63,64]. These viruses (which will collectively be termed HTLV-III for this discussion) have been isolated from over 30% of patients with fully developed AIDS[56], and evidence for viral infection as determined by antibodies to HTLV-III have been detected in nearly 100% of patients with either this syndrome or AIDS-related complex compared to less than 1% of healthy non-risk group controls[67-71]. Moreover, in several cases of transfusion-associated AIDS, HTLV-III infection has been documented in both the transfusion recipient with AIDS and the blood donor, thus providing strong evidence that the transmission of this virus is required for the syndrome to develop[72-75].

The biological characteristics of these viruses observed in vitro has added further support to its causal role in AIDS, since it is selectively tropic for T4 (T-helper) lymphocytes[76] and apears to be cytotoxic for these cells following infection[55]. Recent studies, in fact, have indicated that the virus utilizes the T4 antigen expressed on helper T-lymphocytes as a specific receptor during infection[77,78]. These findings are consistent with the clinical symdrome which, as mentioned previously, is characterized by a progressive and irreversible loss of T4 cells. It is this common abnormality which has been thought to be central to the pathogenesis of AIDS.

However, while the evidence continues to mount that HTLV-III infection is necessary for AIDS to develop, major questions remain concerning the natural history of infection by this virus. Early reports have demonstrated a high prevalence of anti-HTLV-III antibodies in asymptomatic individuals in populations at risk for developing AIDS including 25-65% of healthy homosexual men from areas where AIDS is endemic[79-81], 87% of intravenous-drug users in New York City[82], and 56-72% of persons with hemophilia A[83-85]. From this very large number of individuals with HTLV-III antibodies which by some estimates is in excess of 1 million persons nationally[86], it remains to be determined how many will ultimately develop AIDS or related clinical syndromes and how many are capable of transmitting this virus to other individuals. This problem has been illustrated by the finding that some asymptomatic homosexual men are apparent carriers for HTLV-II which can be cultured from peripheral blood lymphocytes[87,88], semen[88,89], and saliva[87].

The Food and Drug Administration has licensed comercial tests for the detection of HTLV-III antibodies. These tests are used in blood banks to screen units of donated blood for possible HTLV-III contamination in order to reduce the incidence of transfusion-related AIDS which now has affected over 100 individuals. This test will, in addition, provide a means to identify individuals previously infected with HTLV-III[90]. Longitudinal studies of these individuals should provide a better understanding of the consequences of this infection, if any, over time. However, it is important to recognize that tests for HTLV-III antibodies are <u>not</u> "AIDS tests". They do not detect the presence of the retrovirus and, with the present state of knowledge, cannot be used to identify which individuals are likely to transmit the virus or predict who will ultimately develop AIDS. The complex ethical issues surrounding the use and potential misuse of this test will require a clear understanding of these limitations as the HTLV-III antibody tests inevitable gain widespread use[91].

The diagnosis of AIDS continues to require the presence of particular opportunistic infections or malignancies in the setting of an acquired defect in cellular immunity. The discovery that affected individuals have been infected with new virus has provided an important first step in delineating the pathogenesis of immunodeficiency in this tragic epidemic. However, it appears likely that AIDS is but one manifestation of HTLV-III infection. It is possible that the array of immunological abnormalities reviewed earlier for the symposium may ultimately be useful in determining who will develop AIDS among the many individuals infected with HTLV-III. The natural history of HTLV-III infection and the extent to which other host or environmental factors contribute to the evolution of the symdrome are crucial questions facing researchers.

REFERENCES

1. Metroka, C.E., Cunningham-Rundles, S., Pollack, M.S., et al, Ann. Int. Med. 99:585 (1983).
2. Abrams, D.I., Lewis, B.J., Beckstead, J.H., et al. Proc. Am. Soc. Clin. Oncol. (Abstr.) 1:C-183 (1983).
3. Gold, J.W., Sears, C.L., Henry, S., et al., Clinical Res. 31:363A (1983).
4. Ammann, A.J., Wara, D.W., Dritz, S., et al., Lancet 1:956 (1983).
5. Curran, J.W., Lawrence, D.N., Jaffe, H., et al. , New Engl.J. Med. 310:69 (1984).
6. Pitchenik, A., Fischl, M.A., Spira,T.J., et al., J. Am. Med. Assoc. 250:1310 (1983).
7. Rubinstein, A., Sicklick, M., Gupta, A., et al., J. Am. Med. Assoc. 249:2350 (1983).
8. Oleske, J., Minnefor, A., Cooper, R., et al., J. Am. Med. Assoc. 249:2345 (1983).
9. Gottlieb, M.S., Schroff, R., Schanker, H., et al., New Engl. J. Med. 24:1425 (1981).
10. Masur,H., Michelis, M.A., Greene, J.B., et al., New Engl. J. Med. 305:1431 (1981).
11. Siegal, F., Lopez, C., Hammer, G., et al., New Engl. J. Med. 305:1431 (1981).
12. Mildvan, D., Mathur, U., Enlow, R., et al., Ann. Int. Med. 96:700 (1982).
13. Ammann, A., Abrams, D., Conant, M., et al., Clin. Imm. Immpath. 27:315 (1983).
14. Lane, H.C., Masur, H., Edgar, L.C., et al., New England J. Med. 309:453 (1983).
15. Schroff, R.W., Gottlieb, M.S., Prince H.E., et al., Clin. Imm. Immpath. 27:300 (1983).
16. Stahl, R., Friedman-Kien A., Dubin, R., et al., Am. J. Med. 73:171 (1982).
17. Kornfield, H., VandeStouwe, R., Lange, M., et al., New Engl. J. Med. 307:729 (1982).
18. Ryan, D., Betts, R., Cowell, S.,. 23rd Interscience Conf. on Antimicrobial Agents and Chemotherapy (Abstr.) 954 (1983).
19. Fahey, J., Detels, R., Gottlieb, M., et al., New Engl. J. Med. (letter) 308:842 (1983).
20. Fahey, J.L., Prince, H., Weaver, M., et al., Am. J. Med. 76:95 (1984).
21. Rook, A.H., Masur, H., Lane, H.C., et al., J. Clin. Invest. 72:398 (1983).

22. Cunningham-Rundles, S., Michelis, M.A., and Masur, H., J. Clin. Immunol. 3:156 (1983).
23. Kloster, B.E., Clin. Res. 31:347A (1983).
24. Laurence, J., and Kunkel, H.G., Clin. Res. 31:347A (1983).
25. Sell, K.W., Folks, T., Chung Kwon-J.K., et al., New Engl. J. Med. (Letter) 309:1065 (1983).
26. Hersh, E., Mansell, P., Reuben, J., et al., Cancer Res. 43:1905 (1983).
27. Schroff, R.W., Gottlieb, M.S., Prince, H.E., et al., Clin. Imm. Immpath. 27:300 (1983).
28. Ziegler, J.L., Miner, R.C., and Rosenbaum, F., Lancet 2:631. (1982)
29. Hutt-Fletcher, L., Balachandran, N., and Elkins, M.H., J. Exp. Med. 158:2171 (1983).
30. Fauci, A.S., Macher, A.M., Longo, D.L., et al., Ann. Int. Med. 100:92 (1984)
31. Buimovici-Klein, E., Lange, M., Klein, R.J., et al., Lancet 2:344 (1983).
32. Eyster, M.E., Goedert, J.J., Poon, M., et al., New Engl. J. Med. 309:583 (1983).
33. DeStefano, E., Friedman, R.M., Friedman-Kien, J.J., et al., J. Inf. Dis. 146:451 (1982).
34. Zolla-Pazner, S., El-Sadr, W., William, D., et al., N.Y. Acad. Science Conf. on AIDS, in press (1983).
35. Hersh, E.M., Reuben, J.M., Rios, A., et al., New Engl. J. Med. (letter) 308:45 (1983).
36. Naylor, P.H., and Goldstein, A.L., Clin. Imm. Newsletter 4:126 (1983).
37. Essex, M., McLane, M., Lee, T., et al., Science 220:859-862 (1983).
38. Gelmann, E., Popovic, M., Blayney, D., et al., Science 220:862 (1983).
39. Gallo, R.C., Sarin, P.S., and Gelmann, E.P., Science 200:65 (1983).
40. Essex, M.F., McLane, F., Lee, T.H., et al., Science 221:1061 (1983)
41. Ramsey, R., Palmer, E., Feorino, P., et al., Blood 62 (Suppl. 1) 116a (1983).
42. Byrnes, R.K., Chan, W.C., Spira, T.J., et al., J. Am. Med. Assoc. 250:1313 (1983).
43. Iochim, H.L., Lerner, C.W., and Tapper, M.L., J. Am. Med. Assoc. 250:1306 (1983).
44. Abrahm, D., N.Y. Acad. Science Conf. on Aids, in press (1983)
45. Mathur, U., et al., N.Y. Acad. Science Conf. on AIDS, in press (1983).
46. Levine, A.M., Meyer, P.R., Begands, M.K., et al., Ann. Int. Med. 100:7 (1984).

47. Moore, A., Metroka, C., Asch, A., et al., Blood 62 (abstr.) 115a (1983).
48. Volberding, P., N.Y. Acad. Science Conf. on AIDS, in press (1983).
49. Hanto, D.W., Frizzera, G., Purtilo, D.T., et al., Can. Res. 41:4253 (1981).
50. Purtilo, D.T., Paquin, L., Deflorio, D., et al., Sem. in Hematology 16:309 (1979).
51. Center for Disease Control, Morbid. Mortal. Weekly Rep. 31:305 (1982).
52. Scott, G.B., Buck, B.E., Leterman, J.G., et al., New Engl. J. Med. 310:76 (1984).
53. Rubinstein, A., Am. J. Dis. Child. 137:825 (1983).
54. Mayers, m., Bernstein, L., Spigland, I1, et al., 23rd Interscience Conf. on Amtimicrobial Agents and Chemotherapy (Abstr.) 221 (1983).
55. Popovic, M., Sarngadharan, M.G., Read, E., Gallo, R.C., Science 224:497 (1984).
56. Gallo, R.C., Salahuddin, S.Z., Popovic, M., et al., Science 224:500 (1984).
57. Schupbach, J., Popovic, M., Gilden, R.V., et al., Science 224:503 (1984).
58. Barre-Sinoussi, F., Chermann, J.C., Rey, F., et al., Science 224:868 (1983).
59. Vilmer, E., Barre-Sinoussi, F., Rouzioux, C., et al., Lancet 1:753 (1984).
60. Levy, J.A., Hoffman, A.D., Kramer, S.M., et al., Science 225:842 (1984).
61. Ratner, I., Haseltine, W., Patarca, R., et al., Nature 313:277 (1985).
62. Wain-Hobson, S., Sonigo, P., Danos, O., et al., Cell 40:9 (1985).
63. Pescador-Sanchez, R., Power, M.D., Barr, P.J., et al., Science 227:484 (1985).
64. Muesing, M.A., Smith, D.H., Cabradilla, C.D., et al., Nature 313:450 (1985).
65. Luciew, P.A., Poter, S.J., Steimer, K., et al., Nature 312:760 (1984).
66. Arya, S.K., Gallo, R.C., Hahn, B.H., et al., Science 25:927 (1984).
67. Sarngadharan, M.G., Popovic, M., Bruch, L., et al., Science 224:508 (1984).
68. Laurence, J., Brun-Venzinet, F., Schutzer, S.E., et al., New Engl. J. Med. 311:1269 (1984).
69. Safai, B., Groopman, J.E., Popovic, M., et al., Lancet 2:1438 (1984).
70. Kalyanaraman, V.S., Cabradilla, C.D., Getchell, J.P., et al., Science 225:321 (1984).
71. Brun-Vezinet, F., Rouzioux, C., Barre-Sinoussi, F., et al., Lancet 2:1253 (1984).

72. Feorino, P.M., Jaffe, H.W, Palmer, E., et al., Submitted for publication.
73. Feorino, P.M., Kalyanaraman, V.S., Haverkos, H.W., et al., Science 225:69 (1984).
74. Wykoff, R.F., Pearl, E.R., Saulsbury, F.T., et al., New Engl. J. Med. 312:294 (1985).
75. O'Duff, J.F., Isles, A.F., Lancet 2:1346 (1984).
76. Klatzmann, D., Bare-Sinoussi, F., Nugeyre, M.T., et al., Science 225:59 (1984).
77. Dalgleish, A.G, Beverley, P.C.L., Clapham, P.R., et al., Nature 312:763 (1984).
78. Klatzmann, D., Champagne, E., Chamaret, S., et al., Nature 312:763 (1984).
79. Goedert, J.J., Sarngadharan, M.G., Biggar, R.J., et al., Lancet 2:711 (1984).
80. Center for Disease Control, Morbid. Mortal. Weekly Rep. 33:377 (1984).
81. Anderson, R.E., Levy, J.A., Lancet 1:217 (1985).
82. Spira, T.J., Des Jarlais, D.C., Marmor, M. et al., New Engl. J. Med. 311:467 (1984).
83. Ramsey, R.B., Palmer, E.L., McDougal, J.S., et al., Lancet 2:397 (1984).
84. Kitchen, L.W., Barin, F., Sullivan, J.L., et al., Nature 312:367 (1984).
85. Rouzioux, C., Brun-Vezinet, F., Courouce, A.M., et al. Submitted for publication.
86. Landesman, S.H., Ginzburg, H.M., Weiss, S.H., et al., New Engl. J. Med. 312:521 (1985).
87. Groopman, J.E., Salahuddin, S.Z., Sarngadharan, M.G., et al., Science 226:447 (1984).
88. Ho, D., Schooley, R.T., Rota, T.R., et al., Science 226:453 (1984).
89. Zagury, D., Bernard, J., Leibowitch, J. et al., Science 226:49 (1984).
90. Weiss, S.H., Goedert, J.J., Sarngadharan, M.G., et al., J. Amer. Med. Assoc. 253:23 (1985).
91. Goldsmith, M.F., J. Amer. Med. Assoc. 253:173 (1985).

M.I.D.A.S. - AN ON-LINE MICROBIOLOGY INFORMATION SYSTEM

Timothy E. Kiehn

Diagnostic Microbiology Laboratory
Memorial Sloan-Kettering Cancer Center
New York, New York

INTRODUCTION

Computers, so much a part of our society, are now being used by clinical microbiologists as an aid in promptly and accurately delivering and managing specimen results. Within the laboratory structure, attention to microbiology computerization is relatively new and follows computerization of more automated laboratories such as chemistry and hematology. The microbiology laboratory has special needs, such as issuing a series of preliminary results leading to a final result, and thus systems developed initially for other diagnostic laboratories have not produced optimum microbiology additions. However, many vendor and "in-house" developed microbiology computer systems are in operation and descriptions of some of these have been reported[1-5].

In 1981 we decided to install an information system at Memorial Sloan-Kettering Cancer Center (M.S.K.C.C.). By then we had seen several systems in operation, had exchanged ideas about future microbiology requirements with a number of our colleagues, and were aware of our own hospital's experience with a chemistry-hematology system from the Technicon Corporation (LDM-8000). We decided to design our own system and several important concepts were incorporated including on-line delivery of information from technologist operated laboratory terminals directly to terminals located in patient areas, thus employing a "paperless" system. Reduction in the amount of paper associated with a computer system became a very important goal of our plans. Our manual system relied heavily on the transfer of data from one piece of paper to another. This was not only very time consuming but was quite prone to transcription errors. Many of the computerized information systems we saw still had remnants of these manual systems including, in our opinion, continued excessive use of requisitions in the laboratory, worksheets, notes for special requests and protocols, workcards, result cards, mark-sense cards, verification sheets, and automatically generated reports -- many of which were seldom, if ever, read. Thus, we began to think of a system where all information was put immediately into terminals and 'on demand' reports would replace many automatic reports. Maximum use of this on-line system would involve redeployment of work flow in a laboratory operating 168 hours per week. We would begin to observe, record and report test results as soon as the results were available, according to a microbiologic clock, not a "put it in the incubator and read the result the next day" clock.

History

During the 1970's it became apparent to members of the Microbiology Laboratory at M.S.K.C.C. that benefits could be gained from the use of an automated information system. In a laboratory where sophisticated and innovative diagnostic tests were employed, inadequate manual paper systems were still used to assemble the diagnostic results and to deliver these results to the clinicians. These inadequacies became even more apparent as the number of specimens submitted to our laboratory and diagnostic procedures increased, and increased research and development activities put further demands on our data retrieval systems. The advent of several new automated tests suggested even more the potential benefits of computer managed information. In 1981 an administrative decision was made to develop a microbiology information system. I would like to describe the Project Team approach we used for development of our information system and detail a description of that system.

Team Approach

The methodology used for the Microbiology Systems Project was Project Management. The Project Team was made up of representatives of the Infectious Disease Service-Microbiology Laboratory, Information Systems, Hospital Administration and Operational Planning. This team existed throughout the project and in three phases; (I) described the scope of the problem to be investigated, (II) compiled a preliminary system definition and design, and (III) completed the definition and design. At the conclusion of Phase II, a Project Evaluation Report (P.E.R.) was presented to the decision forum, the Information Systems Steering Committee (I.S.S.C.) of the hospital. The P.E.R. described the operations of the current Microbiology Laboratory and its problems, proposed alternatives for data management and recommended a solution.

Project Scope

The project scope included: an examination of all laboratory functions beginning with receipt of a specimen within the laboratory through processing, recording and reporting of information and results. Result reporting had to include rapid delivery of results to clinicians, easy access to results for epidemiologic reports which track infectious occurrences, statistical and managerial reports for laboratory management and external agencies, billing reports for hospital billing systems, and research data for various investigators. Cost effectiveness of the system was to be demonstrated through a structured payback analysis.

While many of the problems identified in the processing of requisitions originate at the point of request, on-line order entry at the nursing units was felt to be best addressed by all laboratories together and thus was eventually determined not to be within the scope of the project.

Current Operations (1981)

The Microbiology Laboratory is part of the Infectious Disease Service in the Department of Medicine. The laboratory is comprised of the following sections: bacteriology, mycology, mycobacteriology, parasitology, serology and virology. We also receive specimens from other institutions and occasionally send specimens outside the hospital. There is also an epidemiology section and we conduct numerous clinical-laboratory research-development studies. In 1981 our staff included 43 full-time and 8 part-time employees, including 34 technologists. At that time the laboratory was staffed from 9 a.m. to 10 p.m. We are now open at all hours, 168 hours per week.

FUNCTIONAL DESCRIPTION

Six segments of the laboratory operation were identified. These included: ordering of tests, evaluation and entry, preparation and processing, work-up, results reporting and data tabulation of results. The following is a brief description of each of the six segments and associated problems. In defining present problems and future needs we gathered information from committees already mentioned and also from other attending physicians, nurses, ward clerks, and research and administrative personnel of M.S.K.C.C.

1. Ordering of tests -- initiated when a clinician requests a laboratory test by noting it on the patient's chart. This request is then entered in the order log at the nurse's station. A laboratory requisition is prepared and the appropriate container

is labelled. Once collected, the specimen is sent to the laboratory. This system includes multiple test requests on the same specimen that requires separate requisitions which can be poorly imprinted and often lack needed information. Incorrect containers may be used and sometimes these containers are delivered to the wrong laboratory.

2. Evaluation and Entry -- the specimen and requisition are checked for acceptability, appropriate notices are sent back to the nurse's station if unacceptable, billing codes are assigned and an accounting copy is submitted to the billing department. Problems included: handwriting of additional requisitions required for multiple tests; manual coding, batching and filing of various copies of the requisition; incomplete, incorrect or illegible information; and manual checking for unnecessary replicate specimens.

3. Preparation and Processing -- specimens are prepared for work-up by the technologist. Problems associated with these functions include labor and error intensive transcription of patient and specimen information on culture plates, tubes and slides; record-keeping of processing time to allow subsequent identification of epidemiology or research data; and parallel tracking of multiple requisitions related to different tests on one specimen.

4. Work-up -- may include: identification of bacteria, fungi and viruses; antibiotic testing; stains for microscopic observation; antibody and metabolite detection tests, parasitic examination, etc. Problems associated with work-up include: poor transfer to results within the laboratory from one area to another, error prone transcription of data to and from work cards, frequent changes in protocols necessitating procedure manual changes, and multiple overlapping research studies causing manual sub-systems for data-tracking and record-keeping.

5. Result Reporting -- preliminary and final results are issued by a paper system and certain urgent results are reported by telephone. Specimens can remain in work-up for approximately 1 to 60 days. Results are not usually available to the clinician between 5:00 p.m. and 9:00 a.m., 125 to 150 phone inquiries are placed to the laboratory each day for results not available due to a lag time for chart insertion of hand written reports, and many preliminary results are not published due to the cumbersome paper system.

6. Data Tabulation -- specimen types and results are tabulated daily, weekly, monthly and annually by epidemiology, management and investigators using manual systems.

There is considerable replication of data tabulation for different groups and difficulty in tabulating data due to a confusing cross-files system.

PRESENT PROBLEMS - SUMMARY

Problems associated with the flow of specimens and information were summarized into three main groups:

A. Poor Communications -- the laboratory's ability to deliver prompt and accurate information to the clinician was constrained by labor intensive procedures. Internal laboratory communications were also limited by the manual operation.

B. Inefficient Operations -- extensive clerical functions associated with the manual paper system occupied a considerable amount of technologist time. Repeated transcriptions of results were time consuming and error intensive.

C. Poor Control of Requisitioning, Collection and Delivery of Specimens -- confusion surrounding which form(s), container(s), test name(s) and which laboratory was appropriate for a given specimen.

COMPUTER SYSTEM - PREFERRED FEATURES

The Project Team defined the preferred features of an information system that would help alleviate the problems listed above.

1. Ordering of tests -- a test information library would define tests provided by each of the clinical laboratories and define appropriate procedures for specimen collection, transportation and processing.

2. Evaluation and Entry -- system would provide option to reject or accept specimen, identify replicate specimens and send appropriate reports back to the requisitioner, automatically send billing information to the billing department, identify special study patients, generate labels and link to a patient information system for receipt of patient demographic information.

3. Work-up -- technologist would work directly with a terminal and enter, immediately, all work-up information. Results could be classified as for internal laboratory use only or for external reporting to the clinician. There would be a capability for interface with automated equipment and procedure protocols would be available and updated via the terminal.

4. Result Reporting -- preliminary and final results would be entered directly into the terminal at the work station by the technologist and be available immediately at terminals throughout the hospital. Individual and chart-reports would be generated. Space occupying hard-copy reports for chart insertion would usually be limited to final reports, due to the emphasis on terminal to terminal use described above.

5. Data Tabulation -- the system would provide both periodic and "on-demand" reports for epidemiology, research personnel and management. Management reports would include inventory reports, significant findings, past-due results, statistical reports and reports for external agencies.

6. Table processing -- we would want to be able to change many listings, in the computer file structure, such as antibiotics, etc., easily within the laboratory, thus reducing reliance on maintenance requirements.

7. Reports on Terminals -- a rapid and simple review process for perusal of results on terminals would be available. For example, if a clinician wanted only blood culture results for a specified period, that request should be simply met.

SYSTEM DECISION

We requested from vendors information pertaining to our system's requirements and asked questions about the ability of their package to fulfill those requirements. We also requested samples of printed reports and system descriptions. Additional site visits were then made to further examine certain systems. After evaluation of these reports we finally decided to develop our own system and we decided that the Microbiology-Infectious Disease Automated System (M.I.D.A.S.) would have an on-line ability for data entry, reporting and inquiry, as well as a batch function for various reports and it would interface with a patient information system and a billing system.

MIDAS FEATURES

I would now like to describe some of the features of the system we have designed. MIDAS is a heavily terminal oriented system with approximately 30 terminals in the Microbiology Laboratory - Infectious Disease Service area and approximately 70 terminals distributed throughout the patient areas. M.I.D.A.S. utilizes the hospital's main-frame IBM 4341 computer. The programming language is ANSI COBOL using both CICS/MVS (command level) and Cullinane's Integrated Data Dictionary/Integrated Data Management System (IDD/IDMS).

Evaluation and Entry

The patient information system provides automatically to M.I.D.A.S. the following information: patient name, location, admitting diagnosis, sex, date of birth and physician of record. Evaluation and entry consists of four phases: entry of patient information, culture information, specimen processing and label generation.

In the patient information mode the accessioner is given an opportunity to enter demographic information, access a patient by name through use of the Soundex system, create a dummy chart number (i.e., for research animal), etc.

Culture information function allows the accessioner to: view the basic demographic and research information for the chart number entered and enter all culture and specimen information necessary to accession a requisition. At this point multiple requests for tests on the same specimen are noted. These codes are present on all screens for that specimen during work-up. Thus, for example, we would know that besides a request for bacteriology, part of a lung tissue specimen is in Mycology, Mycobacteriology and Virology. Entry data could, in addition to standard information, include research project codes and text, special remarks, laboratory memos, antibiotics given to the patient, special information for antibiotic levels and data for metabolite determinations.

The special processing function allows the accessioner to enter reasons for specimen rejection, create rejected and accepted requisition records on the M.I.D.A.S. database, change test/culture information, request additional labels, etc.

A specific number of labels is generated, and the number is determined by the type of test/culture requested.

Preparation and Processing

Once a specimen has been accessioned and labels generated, slides, media and appropriate tests are set up according to various protocols which can be viewed on the terminal screens. General protocol screen information includes whether a Gram stain should be prepared, what agar plates are required, etc.

Specimen Work-Up

Observations and results are classified as either internal (for laboratory observation only) or external (for observation by the requisitioner). Internal and external notations can be changed from one item to the other. This information is entered directly into the terminal via a number of entry screens. These screens are custom designed for each work station and results are entered either by selection from a menu or by entering codes or notations via the key pad. When new information is to be entered, the technologist selects the screen appropriate for that entry. A request can also be made to view all work received at that selected work station (or any other station) on that day. A screen listing all pending work is also available. The pending serology screen lists paired serum from previous tests and results previously entered.

A request for basic work-up screens, made by entry of the

accession number, allows the technologist to view a protocol, view a patient summary, enter a preliminary and/or final finding, enter workcard information, and release findings for verification by the supervisor. Screens include: patient summary, isolate entry, preliminary/final findings, biochemical/sensitivity tests, gram-positive result, gram-negative result, anaerobic result, mycology result, etc.

Batch Negative Reporting

A large number of certain specimens/tests, such as blood cultures, have a negative or no-growth result. The system batches these each day and they are listed on a negative reporting screen. At the end of the incubation period a simple entry of one letter beside each accession number permits release of that result as negative. We decided that a simple, overt gesture should be made rather than an automatic release as negative. If a culture becomes positive it is removed from the negative batch mode and the system places it in the work-up mode.

Verification

All results are verified, by the appropriate person, before they are transmitted to the requisitioner. These results are transferred from work-up to verification by the system and then listed on a verification screen. These results are then viewed individually and accepted for release.

Patient Inquiry

If the clinician does not want to see all microbiology results and is interested in specific test/date information we wanted to provide easy access to this data. The system displays a patient inquiry menu where, after chart number or name are entered, a specific body site or culture/test and specific date or range of dates can be requested. The inquirer is presented with a summary of all cultures/tests requested, with the option of viewing greater detail on any one or more culture/tests desired. For example, all blood cultures for March can be requested, all may be negative and listed on one screen, and thus unncessary time is not needed to search through a number of screens. If positive, as is noted, the specific accession number can be entered and complete information will be displayed for any test.

Results Reporting

Results are viewed on a terminal when a request is made during patient inquiry or findings are printed and delivered to the patient's chart. Easy access to terminals throughout the hospital has eliminated the need for daily ward reports and has reduced the need for printed preliminary results. At the end of each day, final results for each patient, if there are any, are printed. These are organized by test/culture type.

Data Tabulation

Data tabulation utilizes the information gathered in Evaluation and Entry, Work-Up, and Results Reporting to generate reports. These reports are primarily used for epidemiology, laboratory management, and research. Many of these reports are provided on demand and have a variable format. For example, an epidemiologist may request a list of all patients with Pseudomonas aeruginosa isolates from the fifth floor for March, 1984. The system will then retrieve all patients by the given organism, location and time period and list the following additional information for each: date specimen received, chart number, patient name, age, sex, accession number, service, specimen type and final results. Other sorting criteria can be used such as specimen type, organism, time period or service, etc.

Antibiotic reports are produced both periodically and on demand. Trend reports are printed monthly, quarterly and annually. They show the cumulative percent susceptibilities by organism-antibiotic combinations. In addition, specific antibiotic reports can be requested. A requester can supply an organism and a list of antibiotic selections for all specimen types or a specific specimen type such as blood cultures. Additional epidemiologic type information, listed above, will then be provided by the system for each result.

A variety of management and information reports are printed. The following are three examples:

1. A Significant Findings report is printed daily. This report, which is distributed to laboratory management and infectious disease attendings, contains two categories of results. The first lists preliminary or final results of all positive blood and C.S.F. specimens and for each, the chart number, name, location, accession number, date received, specimen type and organism name. A second category includes results as described above for selected specimens such as sterile body sites, virology, etc. This list can be changed as laboratory requirements change.

2. A mycobacteriology log is printed every two months and includes all patients in the past six months who have had positive preliminary or final results for mycobacteriology. The following is printed: accession number; date received; patient name; acid-fast smear results; culture results including date growth was observed on slants or plates, number of colonies, and pigment; inoculation date and identification.

3. The system has a module designed for entry of research information associated with patient specimens. For example, if we are conducting a blood culture study to evaluate a new type of media, research information pertinent to a blood specimen can be entered on a special screen. Each research project is assigned a code and entry of that code calls for that special screen. During the study the requester can assemble study data by selecting criteria by project code, test/culture code, etc. Details are listed, dpending on the request and the type of study.

Table Processing

Complex changes in M.I.D.A.S., as part of a maintenance program, have to be made by Information Systems. However, in the laboratory we are able to easily make minor changes. The table processing function allows us to update, on-line, the following tables: research protocol and project patient, antibiotic identification, biochemical, work-up protocol, organism identification and specimen preparation.

SUMMARY

The system I have described is the result of several years of study and design. A special thanks is in order to our many friends who shared thoughts, both good and bad, about their own systems. Computerization of clinical microbiology laboratories requires planning that varies considerably from other diagnostic laboratories. As we develop and update our systems it will be very important for us to continue this dialogue. The microbiology Computer Users Group, started by George E. Buck at Texas, is a good example of this effort.

REFERENCES

1. Jorgensen, J.H., Holmes, P., Williams, W.L., and Harris, J.L., Computerization of a hospital clinical microbiology laboratory, Am. J. Clin. Pathol. 69:605, (1978).
2. Lawrie, D.J., Elin, R.J., Gill, V.J., Lewis, T. L., McLowry, J.D., and Witebsky, F.G. Microbiology subsystem of a total, dedicated laboratory computer system, J. Clin. Microbiol., 10:861 (1979).
3. Delorme, J., and Cournoyer, G., Computer system for a hospital microbiology laboratory, Am.J. Clin. Pathol. 74:51 (1980).
4. Kyan, K.J., What to look for in a clinical microbiology laboratory computer system, Clin.Microbiol. Newsletter 3:165 (1981).
5. Kunz, L. J., Poitras, J.W., Kissling, J., Mercier, B.A., Cameron, M., Lazarus, C., Moellering, Jr., R.C., and Barnett, G.O. The role of the computer in microbiology, p. 181-183, in "Modern methods in medical microbiology: systems and trends", University Park Bress, Baltimore (1975).

OPPORTUNISTIC MYCOBACTERIAL INFECTIONS

Robert C. Good

Centers for Disease Control
Atlanta, Georgia

INTRODUCTION

Infections with nontuberculous *Mycobacterium* species have been recognized with increasing frequency in recent years, particularly among patient who are immunosuppressed, have prior lung disease, or have undergone invasive procedures and operations. The infections may be self-limited and mild, as in cases of *Mycobacterium marinum* infection, or disseminated and life-threatening, as in some cases of *M. intracellulare* infection. Diagnosis of these infections can present a problem, both because the organisms can be difficult to grow in the laboratory and because they are found in the environment. Furthermore, distinguishing infection from colonization is often difficult. Therapy is complicated because many of the isolates are resistant to antituberculosis drugs, and the results of susceptibility testing with other drugs do not necessarily correlate with therapeutic responses. In addition, the epidemiology of such infections is difficult to study because of the lack of definitive markers.

The tuberculosis case rate in the United States was 11.0 per 100,000 population in 1982[1] and represented a continuing downward trend in new cases being reported. As the incidence of tuberculosis declines, infections due to other *Mycobacterium* species are being reported more frequently. The occurrence of disease due to these species often may be overlooked since they are unexpected. Reports of diptheroids may be made unless an acid-fast stain is used and appropriate culture media are inoculated and incubated for a sufficient period of time.

Tuberculosis is a highly contagious disease which can rapidly spread in an exposed population of healthy persons. Other mycobacterioses are not contagious, and the etiologic agents are usually present in the environment. Therefore, the significance of nontuberculous mycobacteria in clinical specimens must be evaluated carefully. Wolinsky[2] has provided some guidelines which are helpful in establishing whether or not these mycobacterial isolates are a causal agent of disease. Briefly stated, these are as follows: 1) quantity of growth on primary isolation, since moderate to heavy growth rather than a few colonies is indicative of disease; 2) repeated isolation of the same *Mycobacterium* species from the same source; 3) the source of the specimen, since low numbers of mycobacteria may be recovered normally from sterile body fluids and tissues and be indicative of disease; 4) the identification of the isolate may be crucial since certain species are rarely, if ever, associated with disease. A definitive statement on diagnosis has been issued by the American Thoracic Society in their Diagnostic Standards and Classification of Tuberculosis and Other Mycobacterial Diseases[3]. This statement is as follows:

"A definite diagnosis requires (1) evidence, such as an infiltrate visible on a chest roentgenogram, of disease, the cause of which has not been determined by careful clinical and laboratory studies, and (2) either (a) isolation of multiple colonies of the same strain of mycobacteria repeatedly, usually in the absence of other pathogens, or (b) isolation of the mycobacteria from a closed lesion from which the specimen has been collected and handled under sterile conditions--for example, abscess or biopsy tissue."

The currently accepted species of the genus *Mycobacterium* are shown in Table 1. The species shown are from the Approved List of Bacterial Names, 1980[4] updated by the addition of species that have been published since that time[5-10]. The first group includes the strict pathogens *M. tuberculosis*, *M. bovis*, and *M. africanum* (which are collectively referred to as the *M. tuberculosis* complex), *M. ulcerans* and *M. leprae*. Isolation of these organisms is diagnostic of disease; however, the remaining species listed in the table are not strict pathogens but are either opportunistic pathogens or saprophytes. All of the currently recognized photochromogenic species are opportunistic pathogens. These include *M. asiaticum*, *M. kansasii*, *M. marinum* and *M. simiae*. The most often isolated scotochromogenic species is *M. gordonae* which is rarely, if ever, a pathogen. *M. avium* and *M. intracellulare* are grouped together and designated the *M. avium* complex[11]. This complex is the most frequently isolated of the nonphotochromogenic species and is found widely distributed in nature as well as being an opportunistic pathogen. Of the many rapidly growing species, only *M. fortuitum* and *M. chelonae*

Table 1. Currently Accepted Species of the Genus *Mycrobacterium*

Group	Strict or Potential Pathogen	Rarely or Never a Pathogen	
Slowly Growing or Nonculturable Strict Pathogens	*M. africanum*	None	
	M. bovis		
	M. leprae		
	M. tuberculosis		
	M. ulcerans		
Photochromogens	*M. asiaticum*	None	
	M. kansasii		
	M. marinum		
	M. simiae		
Scotochromogens	*M. scrofulaceum*	*M. gordonae*	
	M. szulgai	*M. flavescens*	
	M. xenopi		
Nonphotochromogens	*M. avium*	*M. gastri*	
	M. haemophilum	*M. nonchromogenicum*	
	M. intracellulare	*M. terrae*	
	M. malmoense	*M. triviale*	
	M. shimoidei		
Rapid Growers	*M. chelonae*	*M. agri*	*M. parafortuitum*
	M. fortuitum	*M. aichiense*	*M. obuense*
		M. aurum	*M. phlei*
		M. chitae	*M. pulveris*
		M. chubense	*M. rhodesiae*
		M. fallax	*M. smegmatis*
		M. duvalii	*M. sphagni*
		M. gadium	*M. thermoresistibile*
		M. gilvum	*M. tokaiense*
		M. komossense	*M. vaccae*
		M. neoaurum	
Animal Pathogens	*M. farcinogenes*		
	M. lepraemurium		
	M. microti		
	M. paratuberculosis		
	M. senegalense		

(recommended spelling is chelonae rather than chelonei) are of significance. The animal pathogens have not been found to be etiologic agents of disease in humans.

Many of the Mycobacterium species listed in Table 1 have been isolated throughout the United States. In a survey of 49 participating State and Territorial Laboratories[12] M. tuberculosis was the most common mycobacterial species isolated in 1980, accounting for 65% of the potentially pathogenic isolates and 51% of all mycobacterial isolates. M. avium complex was the second most frequently isolated mycobacterial species accounting for 21% of potentially pathogenic isolates and 16% of total isolates. M. gordonae was the third most commonly encountered species although it is rarely, if ever, associated with disease. This species is commonly found in water and may occur in human specimens as a result of temporary colonization of patients or contamination of laboratory reagents.

Mycobacterial infections caused by species other than the strict pathogens occur principally among patients who are immunosuppressed, have prior lung disease, or have undergone invasive procedures and operations. The characteristics of these mycobacterioses have been presented in the excellent review by Wolinsky[13]. A summation of these characteristics as described by Wolinsky is presented in Table 2 and in the following discussion.

PULMONARY DISEASE

The common species which cause pulmonary disease are M. avium complex and M. kansasii. Other species that may be involved are M. xenopi, M. szulgai, M. simiae, M. scrofulaceum, and M. fortuitum. The average patient is a 48-year-old white male with long standing lung disease and a three-month history of cough, sweats, low fever, and weight loss. Fibrosis and a thin walled cavity in the right upper lobe may be seen on roentgentographs. Sputum will be positive by microscopy and culture. There is no family history of tuberculosis. Treatment of M. kansasii is successful in greater than 90% of cases with isoniazid, ethambutol, and streptomycin for 18 months with rifampin reserved for relapse cases, or an initial treatment regimen of isoniazid, ethambutol, and rifampin for 24 months. Treatment of disease due to the M. avium complex is successful in greater than 70% of patients with 5 to 6 drugs plus resectional surgery after 6 to 8 months of therapy.

A new experimental protocol is being initiated at the Centers for Disease Control to test a new ansamycin which is the only promising drug for the treatment of pulmonary disease due to

Table 2. Opportunistic Infections with *Mycobacterium* Species

Disease Site	Species: Primary	Species: Secondary	Clinical Characteristics and Predisposing Factors	Therapy
Pulmonary	*M. avium* cplx *M. kansasii*	*M. fortuitum* *M. scrofulaceum* *M. simiae* *M. szulgai* *M. xenopi*	48 y.o. white male. Long standing lung disease. 3 month history of coughs sweats, low fever, weight loss. Fibrosis, thin-walled cavity in RUL observed on roentengraph. No family history of TB.	*M. avium* complex - 5 to 6 drugs followed by resectional surgery after 6-8 mos. *M. kansasii* - INH, EMB, SM for 18 mos with RIF reserved for relapse, or INH, EMB, RIF for 24 mos.
Skeletal (Bone, Joint, Tendon)	*M. kansasii* *M. avium* cplx	*M. fortuitum* cplx *M. marinum*	Hand infections following work related trauma. Joints of wrist, elbow or knee diseased. Dental infections. Post-surgical ostemyelitis of sternum.	Surgical drainage and removal of infected synovium and bone. Drugs are rarely helpful except with infections due to *M. kansasii*.
Skin and Soft Tissue	*M. marinum* *M. fortuitum* cplx *M. ulcerans* *M. haemophilum*		Usually follows trauma; however, cutaneous disseminated and multicentric nodular lesions may occur in apparently normal persons.	*M. marinum* infections usually heal spontaneously. Local therapy may include curretage, electrodessication, freezing excision, heat, etc. Drug therapy includes trimethoprim-sulfamethoxazole, tetracycline, minocycline, or EMB/RIF. *M. ulcerans* infections require wide excision and skin grafts, local application of heat or long term therapy with SM and RIF in conjunction with heat and surgery. *M. fortuitum* complex infections are very difficult to treat, but they may respond to amikacin, ethionamide or etythromycin.
Local Lymphadenitis	*M. scrofulaceum* *M. avium* cplx	*M. kansasii* *M. fortuitum*	Child 1-1/2 to 5 y.o.(7 mo.-12 y) usually with enlarged mandibular nodes, but other nodes (pre- or postauricular, parotid inguinal, axillary) maybe involved. Nodal enlargement is usually unilateral, involving groups of nodes. No pain, tenderness, or general symptoms occur. Nodes may soften, rupture or drain. Follows trauma to feet, hands, face or teeth (injection or extraction).	Total excision is treatment of choice. Some reports recommend drug therapy, but multiple drugs would be required for most infections.
Disseminated Disease	*M. avium* cplx *M. kansasii*	*M. fortuitum* cplx *M. scrofulaceum*	Commonly associated with malignancies or other immunosuppressive conditions. Mortality is >70%.	Immunotherapy may be helpful and drugs as above.

*Adapted from Wolinsky (12) with the assistance of Dr. G. P. Kubica.

M. avium complex[14]. Although clofazamine is inhibitory in vitro[15], it has not been proven to be effective in pulmonary disease, presumably because of the low concentration of drug which accumulates in lung tissue.

HUMAN SKELETAL DISEASE

Mycobacterioses involving the skeleton are commonly caused by M. kansasii or M. avium complex. Recently a number of outbreaks, as well as sporadic cases, of sternal infection following cardiac surgery has been due to M. chelonae spp abscessus and M. fortuitum biovar fortuitum. These cases were first seen in 1976, but a common source of infection was often not determined[16-18]; however, in one instance the source was believed to be an ice bath in the operating room[19].

Following trauma, infections of synovia, tendon sheath, or bursa with M. kansasii and M. avium complex may occur. M. fortuitum or M. kansasii may produce disease of the spine, and, as mentioned earlier, the M. fortuitum complex may be associated with postsurgical osteomyelitis of the sternum.

Skeletal disease is treated by surgical removal of the affected area, drainage, or treatment with drugs. In many cases the drugs are not effective. When infections with M. fortuitum complex were first recognized in 1976, we began to identify the members of the complex and look for drugs which would inhibit the organisms. Swenson et al[20] have determined that doxycycline, minocycline, amikacin, and sulfamethoxazole are the drugs most active against M. fortuitum in vitro while amikacin, sisomicin, tobramycin, and erythromycin are the ones most active against M. chelonae. From the lessons learned with tuberculosis, these infections and all other mycobacterioses should be treated with multiple drugs for long periods of time to prevent the emergence of resistant strains.

SKIN AND SOFT TISSUE DISEASE

M. marinum is the cause of swimming pool granuloma and sporotrichoid disease. These infections occur quite often among fishermen and those hobbyists who maintain tropical fish aquaria. M. chelonae and M. fortuitum produce local abscesses following trauma and the Buruli ulcer is caused by M. ulcerans.

M. fortuitum and M. chelonae infections in women have been associated with implantation of protheses for breast augmentation[21]. These infections appear to be sporadic and are not associated with a particular risk factor[22].

M. marinum infections may heal spontaneously or after local treatment, which involves curettage or other such procedures, and therapy with drugs, usually sulfamethoxazole, tetracycline, ethambutol, and rifampin. Infections with M. ulcerans are very difficult to treat. The therapeutic regimen may include wide excision of the ulcer, skin grafts, heat, and long-term streptomycin and rifampin. The treatment for infections caused by the M. fortuitum complex was given earlier.

LYMPHADENITIS

Local lymphadenitis usually is caused by M. scrofulaceum or M. avium complex. Generally it occurs in children 1-1/2 to 5 years old (range 7 months to 12 years). A mandibular node, which is unlateral and painless, is the most common site. A biopsy or aspiration of the node is positive for acid-fast bacilli by microscopy and culture. The lymphadenitis usually follows trauma to the feet, hands, or face, or after dental work has been performed. It is generally 10 times more often due to M. scrofulaceum and M. avium complex than to M. tuberculosis.

If treatment is advisable, it is usually excision of the node although some investigators have reported at least limited response to drugs.

DISSEMINATED MYCOBACTERIOSES

Disseminated mycobacteriosis, usually caused by M. avium complex or M. kansasii, is generally associated with malignancies, especially if the patient is immunosuppressed. The mortality in this disease is greater than 70%. Disseminated disease due to the M. avium complex is common in patients with the acquired immunodeficiency syndrome (AIDS). These infections have been reported for at least 2%-3% of homosexual patients on initial reports to the CDC AIDS Task Force (personal communication, R. Selik, M.D.), but this is underreporting since preliminary reports are filed early before the disease due to M. avium is diagnosed. M. tuberculosis occurs most often in Haitian patients with AIDS. Mycobacterial infections in these immunodeficient patients are represented by masses of acid-fast bacilli which are easily observed in stained sections of lymph nodes, bone marrow, and organs from the patients.

We have identified seven Mycobacterium species isolated from 52 AIDS patients (Table 3). These include single patients with infections due to M. tuberculosis, M. terrae, M. xenopi, M. malmoense, and M. fortuitum. Two patients had infections with M. kansasii, and 45 had infections with M. avium complex. Of the

Table 3. Mycobacterium species isolated from 52 patients with acquired immunodeficiency syndrome (AIDS)

SPECIES	NUMBER OF CASES
M. avium complex	45*
M. fortuitum	1
M. kansasii	2
M. malmoense	1
M. terrae	1
M. tuberculosis	1
M. xenopi	1

* One patient with mixed infection - M. scrofulaceum

45 M. avium complex isolates, 27 were either serotype 4 or serotype 8, or the strains cross-reacted with other types along with 4 and 8. In general, this agrees with the distribution we find in patients with pulmonary disease due to M. avium complex, i.e. serotypes 4 and 8 are most often, but not exclusively, found in cases of disease due to M. avium complex.

Last year we reported 27 cases of bacteremia due to M. chelonae subspecies abscessus and an M. chelonae-like organism among hemodialysis patients[23]. The source of these infections was probably the water used to process dialyzers, either before use or between uses.

Disseminated disease is difficult to treat and results in high mortality. M. avium complex infections are highly resistant to most of the antituberculosis drugs, and new drugs are needed which are active against this organism.

The many manifestations of infections with the rapidly growing mycobacteria have recently been described by Wallace et al[24]. M. chelonae and M. fortuitum were etiologic agents with about equal frequency. Of M. chelonae infections, 80% of isolates were M. chelonae ssp. abscessus and 83% of isolates from infections caused by M. fortuitum were M. fortuitum biovar. fortuitum.

The criteria used to decide that a mycobacterial isolates is truly the cause of disease should be applied to all isolates, and the ATS Diagnostic Standards for Nontuberculous Mycobacterial Disease[4] are reasonable to establish a diagnosis. Mycobacterial infections should be expected more often in certain groups of patients, but a strict interpretation of laboratory results and clinical observations should be applied to avoid needlessly treating these patients with toxic drugs.

Table 4. Serotypes of M. avium complex isolated from 45 patients with acquired immunodeficiency syndrome (AIDS)

SEROTYPE	NUMBER	SEROTYPE	NUMBER	SEROTYPE	NUMBER
1	2	3/8	1	2/4/6	1
2	1	4/8	4/	4/8/21	1
4	9	4/9	1	1/3/4/8	1
5	1	5/9	1		
8	6	6/8	1	Autoag*	5
9	1	8/9	1	NT*	6
13	1	1/8/21	1		

REFERENCES

1. Morbidity and Mortality Weekly Report 32:478, (1983).
2. Wolinsky, E. Revs. Infect. Dis., 3:1025, (1981).
3. American Thoracic Society, Am. Rev. Respir. Dis., 123:343, (1981).
4. Skerman, V.B.D., McGowan, V., and Sneath, P.H.A. Int.J.Syst. Bacteriol., 30:225, (1980).
5. Kazda, J. Int.J. Syst. Bacteriol., 30:77, (1980).
6. Levy-Frebault, V., Rafidinarivo, E., Prome, J.C., Grandry, J., Boisvert, H., and David, H.L. Int.J. Syst. Bacteriol., 33:336, (1983).
7. Tsukamura, M. Int. J. Syst. Bacteriol., 33:336, (1983).
8. Tsukamura, M., Mizuno, S., and Tsukamura, S. Int. J. Syst. Bacteriol. 32:67 (1982).

9. Tsukamura, M., Mizuno, S., and Tsukamura, S., Int. J. Syst. Bacteriol. 33:811 (1983).
10. Tsukamura, M., Mizuno, S., and Tsukamura, S., Int. J. Syst. Bacteriol., 31:263, (1981).
11. Runyon, E.H., Tubercle, 55:235, (1974).
12. Good, R.C., and Snider, D.E., Jr., J. Infect. Dis., 146:829, (1982).
13. Wolinsky, E., Am.Rev. Respir. Dis., 119:107, (1979).
14. Woodley, C.L., and Kilburn, J.O., Am. Rev. Respir. Dis., 126:586, (1982).
15. Gangadharam, P. R., Pratt, P.F., Damle, P.B., and Davidson, P.T., Tubercle, 62:201, (1981).
16. Robicsek, F., Daugherty, H.K., Cook, J.W., Selle, J.G., Masters, T.N., O'Bar, P.R., Fernandez, C.R., Mauney, C.U. and Calhoun, D.M., J. Thorac. Cardiovasc. Surg., 75:91, (1978).
17. Hoffman, P.C., Fraser, D. W., and Hinson, P.L., Am. Rev. Respir. Dis., 117:527, (1978).
18. Hoffman, P.C., Fraser, D. W., Robicsek, F., O'Bar, P.R. and Mauney, C.U., J. Infect. Dis. 143:533, (1981).
19. Kuritsy, J.N., Bullen, M.G., Broome, C.V., Silcox, V.A. Good, R. C., and Wallace, R.J., Jr., Ann. Intern. Med., 98:938, (1983).
20. Swenson, J.M., Thornsberry, C., and Silcox, V., Antimicrob. Agents Chemother., 22:186, (1982).
21. Clegg, H.W., Bertagnoll, P., Hightower, A.W., and Baine, W.B. Plastic Reconstruc. Surg., 72:165, (1983).
22. Cleff, H.W., Foster, M.T., Sanders, W.E., Jr., and Baine, W.B. J. Infect. Dis., 147:427, (1983).
23. Morbidity and Mortality Weekly Report, 32:244, (1983).
24. Wallace, R. J. Jr., Swenson, J.M., Silcox, V.A., Good, R.C., Tschen, J.A., and Stone, M.S., Revs. Infect. Dis., 5:657, (1983).

LABORATORY DIAGNOSIS OF HERPES VIRUSES IN THE IMMUNOCOMPROMISED HOST

Harvey M. Friedman

Hospital of the University of Pennsylvania and Diagnostic Virology Laboratory, The Children's Hospital of Philadelphia, Philadelphia, Pennsylvania 19104

INTRODUCTION

Accurate diagnosis of infections caused by Herpes family viruses has become increasingly important in recent years. In part, this is because effective antiviral chemotherapy is now available for some herpes viruses, but equally important is the impact accurate diagnosis has on reducing dosages of immunosuppressive drugs and on implementing appropriate infection control procedures to prevent nosocomial spread of viral diseases.

In the past decade we have experienced a substantial increase in the incidence of severe herpes virus infections. Advances in cancer chemotherapy have led to more aggressive treatment of patients previously considered incurable. Organ transplantation programs have continued to flourish, in particular, those involving bone marrow, renal or cardiac replacement. A new disease, Acquired Immune Deficiency Syndrome, has appeared in the late 1970's. The net effect of these events is that the hospitalized patient population is likely to consist of one or several persons with markedly depressed immunity. Since viruses of the Herpes family remain latent and tend to reactivate when immunity is suppressed, the above circumstances favor emergence of diseases caused by this group of viruses.

Five viruses comprise the human Herpes family, which include herpes simplex virus (HSV) type 1 and type 2, cytomegalovirus (CMV), Epstein-Barr virus (EBV) and varicella-zoster virus (VZV). Infection with any of these viruses is common in the immunocompromised host; however, as shown in Table 1, the consequences of infection are highly variable, ranging from

Table 1. Herpes Virus Infections in Immunocompromised Patients

Virus	Usual Source of Infection	Common Clinical Manifestations	Rarer Clinical Manifestations
HSV 1	Reactivation of latent virus	Asymptomatic Typical oral mucosal lesions Invasive mucocutaneous disease	Pneumonia Encephalitis Cutaneous or other organ dissemination
HSV 2	Reactivation of latent virus	Typical genital lesions Invasive genital disease	Meningitis Cutaneous or visceral dissemination
CMV	Transplant organs Encephalitis Blood products Reactivation of latent virus	Asymptomatic Fever, Leukopenia Thrombocytopenia Pneumonia, Hepatitis, Nephritis	Chorioretinitis Colonic ulcers
EBV	Reactivation of latent virus	Asymptomatic	Lymphoma If the infection is a primary one, fever, hepatitis, encephalitis may develop.
VZV	Varicella is acquired from patients with chickenpox or shingles	Extensive cutaneous pox Pneumonia Hepatitis	Encephalitis
	Zoster is reactivation of latent varicella virus	Shingles Cutaneous dissemination	Pneumonia Hepatitis Encephalitis

asymptomatic infection to lethal disease.

Although each of the Herpes family viruses can cause disease in immunocompromised patients, certain viruses are common in a particular type of setting. For example, bone marrow transplantation patients have a high incidence of CMV infection (1) while patients with lymphoma are prone to zoster (2). Table 2 describes those herpes virus infections which are most commonly encountered in various immunosuppressive illnesses (2-5). Often, HSV and VZV infections occur within the first 2-4 weeks after immunosuppression with prednisone and azathiprine or after administration of cancer chemotherapy. CMV infections generally develop later, 5-8 weeks into a transplantation course or cancer therapy. Clinical illness with EBV is rare, unless infection occurs in a seronegative patient. This is in contrast to the other Herpes family viruses which often cause disease in the immunocompromised patient after either primary or reactivation infection.

Often the correct viral diagnosis can be made based on the clinical features of infection. For example, chickenpox and shingles have such characteristic appearances that an experienced observer will rarely require confirmation of the clinical impression by laboratory testing. Other viral infections, however, may be less distinctive in their presentation such that laboratory diagnosis is preferred, or even essential, to establish an accurate diagnosis. The clinical features of CMV are so varied

Table 2. Common Herpes Virus Infections in Various Immunosuppressive Diseases

Immunosuppressive Disease	Common Herpes Viral Infections	Comments
Lymphoma	Zoster	5-10% of patients disseminate the infection
Leukemia	Oral HSV	Often locally invasive
AIDS	CMV HSV-genital Zoster	CMV may be lethal and perhaps is a causative factor in Kaposi's sarcoma Genital HSV often locally invasive Zoster heals poorly and may disseminate
Bone marrow, renal, cardiac transplantation	CMV HSV-oral Zoster	CMV pneumonia is particularly severe in bone marrow transplant patients

that laboratory testing is generally required to establish a diagnosis. For HSV the clinical features are often distinctive; however, genital ulcers may be confused with other causes of venereal infections (such as chancroid), oral lesions may have an atypical distribution (for example, mimicking coxsackie virus infections) and cutaneous lesions may be confused with shingles.

Although no firm criteria exist as to which viral infections should be confirmed by laboratory studies, several guidelines can be followed. Patients ill enough to require antiviral chemotherapy should have a confirmed diagnosis. Therapy often is started before viral test results become available; however, a confirmed diagnosis is valuable if either drug toxicities or unexpected complications of the illness develop. A second indication for viral laboratory studies is those situations in which the correct diagnosis is in doubt. A confirmed diagnosis established by viral studies may alter patient management by permitting cancellation of unnecessary tests and medications. Another indication for laboratory diagnosis is the immunocompromised host with viral infection. Often cancer chemotherapy regimens or immunosuppressive drugs can be withheld until the infection clears. Because of the importance of these therapeutic decisions, a laboratory - confirmed diagnosis is preferred.

Currently there are three approaches to viral diagnosis: viral isolation, viral serology and rapid viral detection methods. Each has advantages and disadvantages as described below.

Viral Isolation

This is the "gold standard" against which all other methods are compared for accuracy (6). The types of specimens, culture systems used and description of cytopathology are noted in Table 3. Isolation of a virus from a clinical specimen indicates that the patient has an active infection with that virus. However, to determine whether the virus is actually causing the patient's illness, one must decide if the symptoms are best explained by the virus isolated. In general, specimens taken from diseased organs are most useful. For example, the diagnosis of CMV pneumonia is well established if lung tissue grows only CMV and no other pathogens. However, if a patient with pneumonia does not have a lung biopsy but has CMV in a urine sample, the cause of the pneumonia is far less certain. Therefore, to establish that a virus is the cause of an illness requires correlating viral laboratory studies, clinical symptoms and knowledge of the types of disease caused by the virus.

Several aspects of specimen collection merit emphasis. Most importantly, samples should be transported to the laboratory

Table 3. Viral Isolation

Virus	Usual Source of Specimen	Permissive Cell Culture[1]	Appearance of CPE[2]	Time to CPE	Confirmation of CPE
HSV 1 or 2	vesicle or ulcer from mouth, genitals, skin	MRC-5 HEK	Ballooning	1-3 days	Often not necessary. Can use monoclonal antibodies to type 1 vs. 2.
CMV	throat swab urine, buffy coat, lung tissue	MRC-5	Plaques of round, refractile cells	7-14 days	Often not necessary. Can use IF[3] or ACIF[4] with human sera.
VZV	vesicle swab	MRC-5 HEK	Plaques of round and lysed cells	7-10 days	Often not necessary. Can use IF with animal or human sera.
EBV[5]	throat wash	Cord blood lymphocytes	Transformed cells developed into continuous cell lines.	Up to 28 days for transformation	Use human immune sera by IF or ACIF to confirm presence of EBV antigens.

quickly, since most viruses have a short survival time once outside the body. If transport is delayed, specimens keep best at refrigerator temperatures (4°C). Swabs should be kept moist by placing them in viral transport media, while body fluids, such as urine and spinal fluid, can be transported to the laboratory without special media.

Once a sample arrives at the laboratory it is treated with broad spectrum antibiotics to combat bacterial and fungal contamination. At Children's Hospital of Philadelphia the antibiotics used are vancomycin, gentamicin and amphotericin B (7). Aliquots of the specimen, usually 0.2 ml are then inoculated onto cell monolayers which are grown in 15 cm screw-cap tubes. The cultures are observed by microscopy daily for cytopathology (CPE). If HSV or VZV are suspected based on the clinical features of the illness, cultures are observed for 2 weeks before being discarded as negative. If CMV is suspected, specimens are kept for 4 weeks. A number of factors influence the success rate of viral isolation. These include proper collection techniques, obtaining samples early in the illness when the quantity of virus is maximal, rapid transport to the laboratory, and inoculation of specimens quickly and onto sensitive tissue culture cells.

Viral Serology

Antibody testing is useful to establish a diagnosis of recent infection or to determine the immunity status of a patient or organ donor (Table 4). A diagnosis of recent infection is supported by measuring a four-fold or greater rise in antibody titer in paired serum samples. Alternatively, on a single serum sample detection of viral-specific IgM antibody indicates recent infection. IgM antibody responses occur frequently in primary infection and occasionally in reactivation infection. Currently, IgM assays for Herpes family viruses are not widely available with a possible exception being EBV testing. For this virus a variety of antibodies directed against different antigens can be measured in a single serum sample (8). These include antibodies of the IgG or IgM class against the viral capsid antigen (VCA IgG, VCA IgM), antibodies against early antigen (EA), and antibodies against nuclear antigen (EBNA). The VCA IgG becomes positive during primary infection and remains positive indefinitely. The VCA IgM becomes positive during an active infection returning to negative within a few months. Antibody to EA is often positive for several months showing a diffuse pattern (D) of cytoplasmic fluorescence in primary infection and is positive for years demonstrating restricted pattern (R) of fluorescence in some cancer patients. Antibody to EBNA usually appears 1-2 months after primary infection and remains positive indefinitely. A typical antibody response during primary EBV infection is as follows: VCA IgG, positive, VCA IgM, positive; EA (D), positive; EBNA, negative.

Table 4. Serodiagnosis of Herpes Virus Infections

Virus	Common Indications for Testing	Common Assay Systems[1]	Comments
HSV 1 or 2	To detect titer rise indicative of recent infection.	CF, IAHA	Standard test systems do not distinguish HSV 1 vs 2.
CMV	To detect titer rise indicative of recent infection. To determine immunity status of organ donors and recipients.	CF, IAHA, IF, ACIF, ELISA	Because CMV grows slowly in tissue culture systems, serodiagnosis may preceed viral isolation.
VZV	To detect titer rise indicative of recent infection. To determine immunity status of patient.	IAHA, FAMA, CF, RIA, ELISA	CF test is not sensitive enough to measure immunity. Immunocompromised patients who are seronegative and exposed to varicella should receive prophylactic therapy with high titered immunoglobulin (VZIG).
EBV	To detect anitbodies indicative of recent infection.	IF, ACIF	Serodiagnosis is more commonly used than viral isolation. Monospot test is not reliable for diagnosis of EBV in immunocompromised patients. By measuring antibodies to variety of antigens, the diagnosis can be established on a single serum.

Footnotes to Table 4

1. CF - complement fixation
   IAHA - immune adherence hemagglutination
   IF - immunofluorescence
   ACIF - anti-complementary immunofluorescence
   ELISA- enzyme immunoassay
   FAMA - fluorescent antibody to membrane antigen
   RIA - radioimmunoassay

In the immunocompromised patient antibody responses may be either absent or late in developing. Therefore, in these patients this method of diagnosis is less reliable than in normal hosts. Heterologous antibody responses also can create confusion. For example, patients with HSV infection may develop a four-fold or greater titer rise to both HSV and VZV, or patients with chickenpox and shingles may boost their antibody titers to both VZV and HSV (9). Generally, serologic diagnosis should be used in conjunction with viral isolation rather than as the sole method of diagnosis.

Rapid Viral Diagnosis

In recent years considerable progress has been made in rapid detection techniques. Viruses are either seen using negative staining electron microscopy or viral antigens are detected by immunologic assays in clinical samples before they are inoculated into tissue culture cells. Rapid methods currently in use for Herpes family viruses are presented in Table 5.

With the introduction of monoclonal antibodies, excellent reagents are now available for antigen detection (10). Some of these (HSV 1 and 2) are commercially available, while others are likely to become so in the near future. As investigators develop experience with the use of monoclonal antibodies for rapid viral diagnosis, it has become apparent that the reagents are highly specific but are often less sensitive than polyclonal antibodies. One approach to broaden the range of antigens detected is to include two or more monoclonal antibodies in the testing system (11). In general however, with this family of viruses rapid methods are not as sensitive as viral isolation for establishing a diagnosis (11,12).

Monoclonal antibodies can be used by a variety of assay methods, including immunofluorescence, immunoperoxidase or enzyme immunoassays (12,13). Which of these is best remains to be determined. However, the experience of the laboratory personnel and the equipment which is available will often determine which test is performed by a particular laboratory.

Examination of body fluids, such as urine or vesicle fluid, by the pseudo-replica technique using electron microscopy is another rapid method (14). In general, the virus must be present in high titer (10^4 virus particles/ml) to be detected by this method. The morphology of all Herpes family viruses is identical so that one cannot be distinguished from another by this system.

Rapid detection assays for Herpes viruses are particularly important if the diagnosis is in doubt or if the infection can be treated with antiviral drugs. For example, patients with

Table 5. Rapid Diagnosis of Herpes Family Viruses

Virus	Rapid Methods[1]	Usual Samples	Comments
HSV 1 or 2	IF, IPA, EM, ELISA Tzank preparation,	Vesicle or ulcer scrapings. Brain or other organs.	Most useful for encephalitis.
CMV	IF, IPA, ELISA, EM, DNA hybridization, histopathology	Lung tissue urine buffy coat	Sensitivity of the rapid assays are not well established.
VZV	IF, IPA, ELISA, EM Tzank preparation	Vesicle scrapings or fluid	Diagnosis can usually be made by clinical evaluation.
EBV	none	—	—

Footnotes: [1] IF - immunofluorescence; IPA - immunoperoxidase; ELISA - enzyme immunoassay EM - electron microscopy

encephalitis who have focal neurologic deficits often have HSV as the cause of their illness. Brain tissue, obtained by biopsy, can be examined by rapid methods (immunofluorescence, immunoperoxidase or electron microscopy) to establish the cause and help guide therapy. Another example is the immunocompromised patient with fever. CMV is often considered in the differential diagnosis but may require 10-21 days (or longer) for growth in tissue culture. Although a variety of rapid methods to detect CMV are listed in Table 5, at present none is very sensitive with the possible exception of DNA hybridization. Recently, using radiolabeled CMV DNA fragments as probes, several investigators have detected CMV in body fluids or tissue samples (16-18). Although the sensitivity of this assay is probably not as good as viral isolation, it is specific and the detection is much more rapid (2 days or less). As methodology for this new assay system improves, it may become a practical and widely available technique (19).

Many infections caused by the herpes family of viruses can be diagnosed with accuracy based on the clinical features of the illness. However, for those infections requiring laboratory confirmation, viral isolation remains the most reliable method for HSV, CMV and VZV. For EBV serologic diagnosis is preferred. In the past decade, major advances have occurred in the field of rapid viral diagnosis. Reagents and technology have improved remarkably and the outlook for the future remains promising for continued progress in this discipline.

REFERENCES

1. Neiman, P.E., Reeves, W., Ray, G., Flournoy, N., Lerner, K.G., Sale, G.E., and Thomas, E. D., J. Infect. Dis. 136:754 (1977).
2. Dolin, R., Reichman, R. C., Mazur, M.H., and Whitley, R. J., Ann. Intern. Med. 89:375 (1978).
3. Betts, R. F., and Hanshaw, J. B., Ann. Rev. Med. 28:103 (1977).
4. Muller, S. A. Herrmann, E. C., and Winkelmann, R. K., Am. J. Med. 52:102 (1972).
5. Grose, C., Henle, W., and Howritz, M. S., So. Med. J. 70:1276 (1977).
6. Schmidt, N. J., in Diagnostic Procedures for Viral, Rickettsial and Chlamydial Infections. Lennette, E.H., Schmidt, N.J. (eds) American Public Health Assoc. Washington, D. C. p. 65 (1979).
7. Forrer, C. B., Blahy, Om M., Maitico, A. L., Campos, J. M., and Friedman, H. M., J. Clin. Microbiol. 16:295 (1982).
8. Henle, W., Henle, G. E., and Horwitz, C. A., Hum. Pathol. 5:551 (1974).
9. Forghani, B., Schmidt, N. J., and Dennis, J., J. Clin.

Microbiol. 8:545 (1978).
10. Nowinski, R. C., Tam, M. R., Goldstein, L. C., Stong, L., Kuo, C-C, Corey, L., Stamm, W. E., Handsfield, H. H., Knapp, J. S., and Holmes, K., Science 219:637 (1983).
11. Goldstein, L. C., Corey, L., McDougall, J.K., Tolentino, E., and Nowjinski, R.C., J. Infect. Dis. 147:829 (1983).
12. Schmidt, N. J., Dennis, J., Devlin, V., Gallo, D., and Mills, J., J. Clin. Microbiol. 18:445 (1983).
13. Yolken, R.H., in New Developments in Diagnostic Virology: Current Topics in Microbiology and Immunology. Backmann, P.A. (ed.) Springer-Verlag. Berlin 104:177 (1983).
14. Macris M. P., Nahmias, A.J., Bailey, P.D., Lee, F.K., Visintine, A. M., and Barann, A. W., J. Virol. Methods 2:315 (1981).
15. Goldstein, L.C., McDougall, J., Hackman, R., Meyers, J. D., Thomas, E. D., and Nowinski, R.C., Infect. Immun. 38:273 (1982).
16. Chou, S., and Merigan, T.C., N. Engl. J. Med. 308:921 (1983).
17. Spector, S.A., Rua, J.A., Spector, D.H., and McMillan, R., 23rd Interscience Conference on Antimicrobial Agents and Chemotherapy. Las Vegas. Oct 24-26, 1983, Abstract 914 (1983).
18. Marlowe, S., Watkins, P., Kowalsky, P., Hirsch, M., and Crumpacker, C., 23rd Interscience Conference on Antimicrobial Agents and Chemotherapy. Las Vegas. Oct 24-26, 1983, Abstract 312 (1983).
19. Brigati, D. J., Myerson, D., Leary, J. J., Spalholz, B., Travis, S. Z., Fong, C.K.Y., Hsiung, G.D., and Ward, D.C., Virology 126:32 (1983).

HERPESVIRUS INFECTIONS IN THE IMMUNOCOMPROMISED HOST: DIAGNOSIS AND MANAGEMENT

Richard J. Whitley

Departments of Pediatrics and Microbiology
University of Alabama School of Medicine
Birmingham, Alabama

INTRODUCTION

Infection is a common complication in the treatment of patients with cancer, and, as such, remains the major cause of death[1]. Impairment of host defenses can be a consequence of either the therapeutic modalities designed to bring the malignancy under control or the primary disease. As a consequence, normal resident microbes of the skin, gastrointestinal tract, and the environment as well as those which are already latent in the body, namely the human herpesviruses, can assume enhanced pathogenicity. The importance of early recognition of infection, regardless of microbial etiology, its prompt and specific diagnosis, and the approriate intervention with antimicrobial therapies are of paramount importance in the successful management of all immunocompromised patients.

One consequence of modern medical management of human malignancies with the widespread utilization of cytolytic and cytotoxic drugs is that the risk/benefit factor is tilted toward increased pathologic potential for many of the human herpesviruses. Consequently, there is an increasing number of individuals who suffer from exaggerated herpetic infections that often approach life-threatening proportions. A need exists to understand the pathogenesis of these infections, develop rapid diagnostic procedures, and implement proper therapy without endangering the patient. This review will focus on three of the major human herpesviruses which cause significant diagnostic and medical problems in the immunocompromised host: cytomegalovirus, varicella-zoster virus, and herpes simplex virus. Particular emphasis will be placed on therapeutic approaches to the management of infections caused by herpesviruses.

Herpesvirus infections in the normal host are usually benign with the few exceptions of herpes simplex encephalitis, neonatal herpes simplex virus infection, and congenital cytomegalovirus infection. However, in the immunocompromised host diseases which are normally benign and, for the most part a nuisance, can take on life-threatening proportions. These resulting diseases are of importance from a clinical standpoint and are summarized in Table 1.

Table 1
HERPESVIRUS INFECTIONS IN THE IMMUNOCOMPROMISED HOST

HERPES SIMPLEX	- CHRONIC PROGRESSIVE MUCOCUTANEOUS INFECTIONS
	- ESOPHAGITIS
	- HEPATITIS
	- PNEUMONITIS
VARICELLA-ZOSTER	- PENUMONITIS
CHICKENPOX	- ENCEPHALITIS
SHINGLES	- HEPATITIS
EPSTEIN-BARR VIRUS	- PROTRACTED MONONUCLEOSIS SYNDROME

The most common of the herpesvirus infections are those caused by herpes simplex virus which can result in chronic progressive mucocutaneous infections, esophagitis, hepatitis, or pneumonitis, and rarely, death. Varicella-zoster virus infections are associated with, in its primary form, chickenpox, or its recurrent form, herpes zoster or shingles. Regardless of primary or recurrent infection, pneumonitis, encephalitis, and hepatitis occur in a significant proportion of patients who are immunocompromised. Cytomegalovirus is most frequently associated with pneumonitis in the immunocompromised host, particularly in bone marrow transplant recipients where mortality is exceedingly high. Furthermore, these viruses have been associated with graft rejection in renal transplant recipients. The clinical manifestations of Epstein-Barr virus in the immunocompromised host is not well understood. The first three viruses will be considered separately.

HERPES SIMPLEX VIRUS INFECTIONS

Herpes simplex virus infections in the immunocompromised host can be unusually severe, slow to heal, and associated with prolonged viral shedding[2-6]. Recurrent herpes simplex virus infections in these patients are frequently associated with intraoral and labial pain, resulting in anorexia and often, facial disfigurement[2-5]. Renal, bone marrow, and cardiac transplant recipients are at

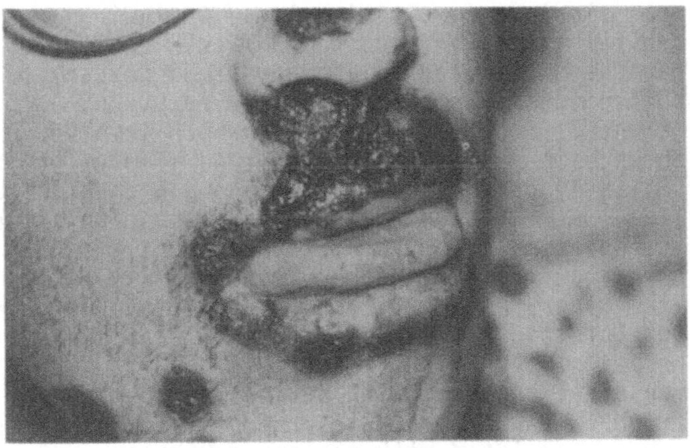

Fig. 1. Progressive mucocutaneous herpes simplex infection in immunocompromised host.

particular risk for increased severity of herpes simplex virus infections. Otherwise benign, recurrent infections of the lip take on an exaggerated course. An example of exaggerated infection is displayed in Figure 1.

In contrast to herpes simplex virus infections of the normal host, healing in the immunocompromised host takes place over a prolonged period. As Spruance and colleagues have reported, healing in the normal host begins rapidly after the appearance of vesicles and parallels the decline in the quantity of virus recovered from these lesions[7]. Generally, virus can no longer be detected after 120 hours and healing for the most part is complete by seven to ten days. In contrast, infection is prolonged in many immunocompromised patients. Obviously, some immunocompromised patients lose virus from lesions, have no pain, and heal completely during the first ten days while others continue to excrete virus and fail to heal even six to eight weeks after the onset of lesions. The size of the lesions appears to be a major determinant of healing. Namely, those individuals with larger lesions require a longer time to heal than those with smaller lesions[8]. Interestingly, many immunocompromised hosts excrete herpes simplex at multiple sites, including mouth and lip, mouth and genital tract, and mouth and face. Dual sites of viral excretion have been obtained in as many as 30 percent of immunocompromised patients suffering from recurrent herpes simplex virus infections[8]. Progressive disease which involves visceral organs is an uncommon complication. Herpes simplex esophagitis, often concomitantly diagnosed with *Candida albicans* infection, has been reported[9]. As experience with organ transplantation increases, herpes simplex pneumonitis and hepatitis have appeared to increase in the frequency of occurrence[4,10,11]. Organ transplant recipients are particularly prone to develop herpes simplex virus infections. As summarized by Pass and colleagues, recurrent herpes simplex virus infections occurred in 75 percent of renal transplant patients with antibodies to herpes simplex virus infection[2]. In these studies, herpes simplex virus infections were associated with prolonged viral shedding, but, as noted previously, in the absence of the appearance of visceral complications. When these infections occur, they generally do so between two and four weeks after transplantation, a time at which immunosuppressive therapy with prednisone and imuran is greatest[9,12]. In the case of other diseases such as leukemia or lymphoma, the reactivation rate after treatment is not as well defined; however, it appears to be similar to that encountered following organ transplantation[13].

DIAGNOSIS

Isolation of herpes simplex viruses, either type 1 or 2, in tissue culture remains the standard for diagnosis. Fortunately, these viruses grow in a wide variety of tissue culture cells. Commonly employed cell lines include primary rabbit kidney, human embryonic, human amnion cells, human diploid fibroblast and African green monkey kidney cells. One monkey kidney cell line

(Vero cells) may be the most sensitive for isolation of herpes simplex virus in tissue culture. After inoculation of clinical swab specimens clarified at 600g into susceptible cell lines, cytopathic effect is sought daily. The most common form of cytopathic effect is the appearance of cytoplasmic granulation followed by ballooning of cells, 'rounding' and lytic degeneration. An alternative type of cytopathic effect is the formation of multinucleated giant cells which result from virus induced fusion of cell membranes. The specific virus type can be determined utilizing principles of monoclonal antibody staining of virus isolates or restriction endonuclease analysis of viral DNA.

Alternative methods of laboratory diagnosis include electron microscopic examination of scrappings of vesicular lesions or fluid obtained directly from the vesicle. Similarly, cell scrappings of lesions can be stained with monoclonal antibodies to herpes simplex virus proteins for demonstration of the presence of viral antigens. This modality of diagnosis, although not currently marketed, will likely be approved by regulatory authorities within the next six months.

Serologic assays have been most helpful in the diagnosis of primary infections but are presently of little value in establishing the nature of a recurrent episode of infection. The available serologic assays include: immunofluorescence, complement fixation, neutralization, hemadsorption, solid phase radioimmunoassay, and ELISA. The diagnostic approaches to herpes simplex virus infections have been well reviewed by Dr. Rawls[14].

THERAPY

The severe and progressive nature of herpes simplex virus infections of immunocompromised patients has prompted therapeutic trials with a variety of antiviral agents. Medications have been administered by intravenous, oral, and topical routes. The two major compounds which have been studied for the treatment of these infections are vidarabine, a drug which is an inhibitor of both host cell and viral replication, and acyclovir, a drug specifically activated by herpes simplex virus thymidine kinase. Acyclovir then acts as a selective inhibitor, following further phosphorylation by cellular kinases, at the level of herpes simplex virus DNA polymerase. It is this latter drug which has been evaluated extensively. In a study of 97 immunocompromised patients with progressive herpes simplex virus infections, intravenous acyclovir therapy at a dosage of 250mg/m^2 over a one hour period every eight hours for seven days or placebo resulted in a significantly beneficial effect for drug recipients[15]. Forty-six of these patients were bone marrow transplant recipients while 13 were renal or cardiac transplant patients and 38 were immunosuppressed for other reasons. Acyclovir therapy for the total population decreased virus shedding times from 16.8 to 2.8, pain from 13.1 to 8.9, scabbing from 13.5 to 9.3, and total healing from 20.1 to 13.7 days. All events were accelerated at a statistically significant level $p<0.05$ for each parameter (two-tailed test). When patients were segregated according to underlying illness, those individuals who were immunocompromised for reasons other than bone marrow transplantation derived even greater benefit for loss of pain and time to total scabbing when compared to their counterpart bone marrow transplant recipients, $p<0.02$ (two-tailed test for both parameters). In this trial, there was no evidence of toxicity.

These studies have been extended to a study of topically applied acyclovir to apparent cutaneous lesions. This trial included 63 individuals who were renal transplant recipients, leukemics or were immunocompromised for other reasons. Topical application of acyclovir accelerated clearance of virus from lesions, loss of pain, and time to total healing by an average of five to nine days for each parameter. The size of the lesion is one factor which influenced the total events of healing, The beneficial effects of topically applied acyclovir in this study population resembled that encountered with intravenous therapy. Obviously, however, the beneficial effects were dependent upon the availability of lesions for topical application of medication.

Saral and colleagues developed a novel approach for the prevention of herpes simplex virus infections in high risk populations[16]. They demonstrated that acyclovir therapy could be administered prophylactically and lead to prevention or amelioration of severe herpesvirus infections following bone marrow transplantation. Nevertheless, in this study as in the studies of Wade and Meyers, the discontinuation of parenteral antiviral therapy led promptly to recurrences which required readministration of parenteral antiviral therapy[15,17].

Vidarabine therapy has been shown to be useful for the treatment of herpes simplex encephalitis and neonatal herpes simplex virus infections[18-21]. It has been studied in the immunocompromised host for herpes simplex virus infections, utilizing a cross-over study design. However, because of the study design and exceedingly long period of infection pretherapy, the beneficial effects of therapy with this medication for mucocutaneous herpes simplex infection were more limited when compared to other herpes simplex virus infections. Specifically, patients who received vidarabine demonstrated accelerated defervescence, loss of pain, and in patients over forty years of age, clearance of herpes simplex virus type 1; however, there was only limited evidence for enhanced total healing[22].

The treatment trials of progressive herpes simplex virus infections of the immunocompromised host elucidate the difficulties encountered in managing patients with prolonged and chronic viral infection. Because of the prolonged nature of infection, the time frame for effective therapy is broader and should allow for easier demonstration of clinical benefit. Clearly, a better approach would be the prevention of herpes simplex virus infections in the immunocompromised host rather than the treatment after the fact.

VARICELLA-ZOSTER VIRUS INFECTIONS

Varicella-zoster virus infections in the immunocompromised host pose significant hazards of both morbidity and mortality. This is particularly true for individuals developing chickenpox as the infection takes on proportions not evident in the normal host. The natural history of chickenpox in the immunocompromised host is associated with prolonged lesion formation. As in the normal host, the rash begins centrally and spreads peripherally; however, the lesions tend to be larger and more numerous. It is not uncommon for the lesions to have hemorrhagic bases with large purpuric spots surrounding them. New lesions continue to form for a period of approximately ten days with fever persisting as long as two weeks after the onset of infection[25]. The time to complete scabbing and resolution of disease is approximately two-fold that of the normal host.

When immunocompromised children are evaluated prospectively for the appearance of complications in the absence of therapy, of thirty-six children, ten developed life-threatening disease and six died.[25,26]. These individuals had lymphoproliferative malignancies and required continuous chemotherapy, being at greatest risk for progressive visceral involvement and death.

The largest historical survey of chickenpox in children with lymphoproliferative malignancies and solid tumors was performed by Feldman at St. Jude's Hospital during the period of 1962-1973[23]. Progressive checkenpox occurred infrequently in children who did not receive chemotherapy for induction or relapse. Yet, one-third of the children who received cancer chemotherapy developed progressive disease with involvement of multiple organs including the lungs, liver, and/or central nervous system. Pneumonitis was the most severe complication. Feldman reached the conclusion that if chemotherapy was terminated five days prior to the onset of chickenpox, the frequency of progression to severe illness was decreased. Observations by other investigators of asthmatic children receiving prednisone (up to 15mg/day) do not support increased risk in subpopulations of these patients[24].

The recurrent form of varicella-zoser virus infection is shingles, an infection complicated by an underlying malignancy. Disease is exaggerated with prolonged periods of vesicle formation and time to total healing. The median time to total cessation of new vesicle formation, total pustulation, and scabbing in a group of 59 untreated immunocompromised patients was 8, 9, and 18 days, respectively. Thus, the natural history is extended by approximately one week when compared to the normal host[27].

Those patients at greatest risk for developing herpes zoster with visceral complications are individuals suffering from Hodgkin's disease and non-Hodgkin's lymphoma. Cutaneous dissemination can occur in 40 percent of these patients and visceral involvement in 10 percent. Death occurs in 4 to 8 percent of patients, overall[27].

DIAGNOSIS

As with herpes simplex virus, unequivocal confirmation of diagnosis is possible only through isolation of virus in susceptible tissue culture lines or the demonstration of seroconversion in the seronegative individual by serial antibody assessment. A rapid diagnostic impression can be obtained by scrapping the base of lesions in an attempt to demonstrate the presence of intranuclear inclusion bodies and multinucleated giant cells by Tzanck smears. These changes are not pathognomonic for varicella-zoster virus infections and require differentiation from the other herpesviruses. Vesicles should be aspirated at the bedside with a tuberculin syringe containing viral transport media and then inoculated into susceptible cell lines. Such cell lines include human embryonic skin muscle tissue or foreskin fibroblasts. Although ctyopathic effects indicative of varicella-zoster virus infections can appear in 48-72 hours, it is more likely to appear approximately seven to ten days after inoculation of the clinical specimens into tissue.

Serologic assessment of patients with VZV infection has focused historically on utilization of the complement fixation antibody assay. More contemporary approaches have included immunofluorescence, a fluorescent membrane antigen assay (FAMA), complement dependent neutralization immune adherence hemagglutination (IAHA) and ezyme-linked immunosorbent. These assays have been reviewed in detail[28]. The value of serology in defining shingles is less useful than for primary infection caused by varicella-zoster virus infection.

TREATMENT

Clinical Management of Varicella

Prevention. Because the immunocompromised child is at risk for developing progressive varicella, two potential modalities of prevention are immune prophylaxis and vaccination. Ross has studied the effect of serum gamma globulin at varying dosages in 242 children exposed to chickenpox and given gamma globulin within 72 hours[29]. The results were compared to data derived from 209 children who served as untreated controls. Higher dosages of immune serum globulin resulted in a significantly decreased total vesicular count. Children who formed less than 20 lesions accounted for approximately 40 percent of the immune serum globulin group as compared to only 1 percent of those in the control group.

Subsequently, a field trial was performed to assess the value of high titered immune globulin for the prevention of disease[30]. This globulin product has become known as zoster immune globulin, ZIG, and is derived from adults suffering from recent herpes zoster. In these patients, the quantity of antibodies was found to be significantly higher than that following the primary infection of chickenpox. In double-blind, placebo-controlled studies of six families, the recipients of ZIG failed to develop evidence of chickenpox while the controls acquired disease[30]. Thus, the conclusion was that ZIG appeared to prevent infection when given to healthy children shortly after exposure.

This study served as a foundation for more complex trials which were performed in immunocompromised children at high risk. Safety and tolerance studies performed following the administration of 5 ml of ZIG to high-risk household contacts of children with chickenpox demonstrated the ameliorative and/or protective effects of this product[31,32]. The administration of ZIG did not unequivocally prevent disease but simply modified the disease course. Its utilization has become increasingly widespread.

For true effectiveness, ZIG must be administered within 72 hours of contact and only to individuals at extreme high-risk. It is available for individuals with underlying diseases of leukemia or lymphoma, congenital or acquired immunodeficiency, active immunosuppressive therapy, or the newborn of a mother with chickenpox who developed disease within four days of delivery. For purposes of ZIG administration, close exposures is defined as either a household contact, indoor contact of greater than one hour with a playmate or a hospital contact on the same ward. There should be no prior history of chickenpox and the age of the patient should be less than 15 years[33]. Zoster immune globulin can be obtained for immunodeficient children through the local Red Cross offices and hospital pharmacies.

Vaccination. Only recently has a live attenuated vaccine been developed for prevention of chickenpox in high risk groups, particularly through the efforts of Takahashi and coworkers[34,35]. Results from these trials were summarized in 1975[34]. In a series of studies, these investigators examined the effect of vaccination on the transmissability of VZV in a childrens' hospital ward among susceptible children. The patients on this ward suffered from a variety of diseases, including nephrotic syndrome, nephritis, bacterial meningitis, and hepatitis. With vaccination, side effects were minimal; only two children developed a minimal rash 10-14 days after vaccination[35]. This study demonstrated prevention of transmission within a high risk group.

Subsequently, a series of trials have been performed in immunocompromised children to determine the protective efficacy of this attenuated VZV vaccine. In these studies, vaccine recipients seroconverted with approximately 8 percent developing a mild rash 10-14 days after immunization[36]. The follow-up of these vaccine recipients two years after immunization demonstrated persistence of immunity in 50 of 51 original vaccinees with apparent protective immunity in most children who had received the vaccine[37]. These landmark studies were performed in immunocompromised children who no longer received chemotherapy. Further studies have been conducted in children whose chemotherapy has not been suspended. In this subgroup of patients, the incidence of side effects and the appearance of rash suggestive of varicella occur frequently, indicating a degree of concern for the status of chemotherapy at the time of immunization[38]. It appears as though the vaccine is protective but not without risk. An unknown entity at this time is whether the administration of vaccine will change the subsequent natural history of herpes zoster or predispose the immunocompromised child to severe forms of herpes zoster as are encountered in other immunosuppressed patients.

In the United States, a multi-center study is in progress to further elaborate on the protective effects of vaccination. These studies are being conducted by Dr. Ann Gershon and are sponsored by the National Institute of Allergy and Infectious Diseases. In these studies a two immunization regimen is being utilized in order to potentially circumvent the problem of waning antibody.

Similar concerns exist regarding the universal administration of this vaccine to the normal host. If universal vaccination is to be employed, it would be important to determine whether such a procedure would change the epidemiology of VZV infections, allowing for a larger number of cases of chickenpox during adulthood at which time the infection might be more severe. It is inconceivable to think that a live-attenuated VZV vaccine will prevent reactivation of virus later in life, given the propensity of this virus to establish latency and recur.

Antiviral Treatment. Because of the recognized complications of varicella, several experimental antiviral treatments have been attempted in immunocompromised subjects. Historically, the first of the therapeutic trials employed cytosine arabinoside, a drug which failed because of a low therapeutic index (ratio of efficacy to toxicity).[39-43]. The first successful antiviral chemotherapy trials conducted in the United States for the management of chickenpox in the immunocompromised host have utilized the drug adenine arabinoside or vidarabine. In carefully controlled investigations of 34 immunocompromised patients performed by the NIAID Collaborative Antiviral Study Group, a dosage of 10mg/kg/day led to the observation that treated patients ceased forming new lesions and defervesced more rapidly than their placebo counterparts[25]. Most importantly, the treated patients had a significantly lower incidence of life-threatening complications which appeared after the onset of therapy, 53 percent in placebo versus 5 percent in drug recipients, $p<0.01$ (Fischer exact test)[25]. Thus, when therapy is instituted within 72 hours of the onset of chickenpox in the immunocompromised host, it can beneficially influence the outcome of this disease. A similar study model was employed for the evaluation of acyclovir and reported by Prober and colleagues[44]. In that 20 patient trial, therapy had no effect on cutaneous healing or fever; however, the administration of acyclovir did decrease the development of pneumonitis from 45 percent to 0 percent. Both drugs appear to be without significant toxicity in these patients.

Interferons are a series of naturally occurring small molecular weight glycoproteins which, among other functions, act as a host defense to viral infection. High titers of interferon have been found in vesicle fluid from patients with varicella at the termination of illness, suggesting that interferon may play a role in the control of this disease[45]. Arvin reported that high dosages of interferon decreased the frequency of visceral complications and prevented progressive disease in children with varicella[26]. The dosage of interferon used in these studies was 30×10^6 IU administered intramuscularly daily for five days. These interferons were produced by Dr. Kari Cantell in Finland from leukocytes harvested and challenged for interferon production. To date no studies have reported evaluations of recombinant DNA interferons alone or in combination with antiviral agents for the management of varicella in high risk populations, yet these studies are in progress in the United States. Data will likely be forthcoming in the near future.

Clinical Management of Herpes Zoster

Antiviral therapy. Specific therapeutic measures have been developed for treatment of herpes zoster in the immunocompromised host. First, however, excellent skin care with Domeboro soaks is essential. Administration of steroids may be useful[46] but may also prolong healing within the dermatome[47]. Obviously, the high risk patient with lymphoproliferative malignancy has the greatest need for parenteral antiviral therapy. At the present, those therapies have been evaluated in large controlled studies and shown to be useful. In two studies, vidarabine has been shown to accelerate the events of cutaneous healing, namely cessation of new vesicle formation, time to total pustulation, and scabbing, as shown in Figure 2. Furthermore, therapy within 72 hours of onset

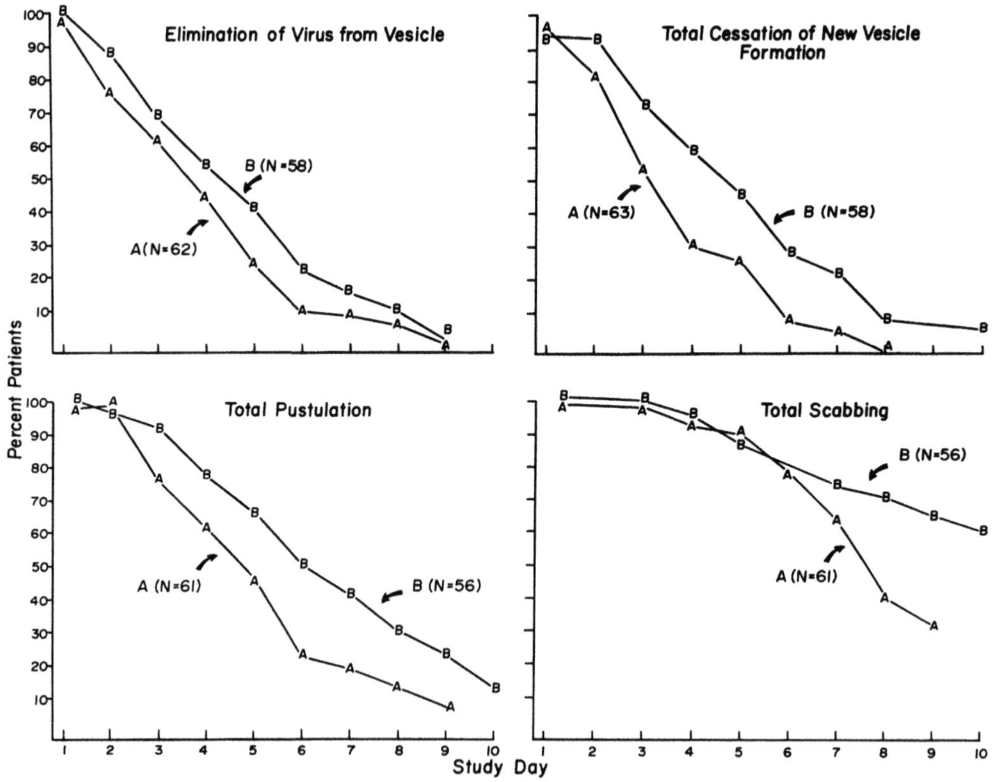

Fig. 2. Herpes Zoster: Events of Cutaneous Healing

prevents progression of lesion formation within the dermatome and allows gradual regression of the disease in the area involved[47]. The most important advantage of administration of vidarabine to immunocompromised patients is the reduction of visceral complications from an overall frequency of 19 percent to 5 percent. Of the 58 placebo recipients with herpes zoster, eleven had significant complications which included encephalitis (three patients, 5 percent), hepatitis (three patients), and uveitis leading to blindness (three patients). Thus, early vidarabine therapy administered within 72 hours of lesion formation is effective in preventing complications and accelerating healing. These benefits can be achieved at a dosage of 10 mg/kg/day administered in standard intravenous solutions at a concentration of 0.5 mg/ml over 12 hours for five days.

A common problem encountered with vidarabine treatment of the immunocompromised host with herpes zoster is the necessity for hospitalization and intravenous drug administration over a prolonged time. Vidarabine is a relatively insoluble drug which requires continuous administration over 12 hours. Hopefully, the development of antiviral medications which can be administered by mouth will obviate the need for hospitalization of these patients. There is no evidence to suggest that either zoster immune globulin or zoster immune plasma will alter the expression of disease once present.

The second therapeutic modality which has been evaluated is the administration of interferon which has been employed successfully in a dose escalating study of 90 patients with herpes zoster and an underlying malignancy[48]. In this study, performed by Merigan and colleagues, administration of interferon at a dosage of 1-2 x 10^6 IU/kg intramuscularly resulted in decreased progressive vesicle formation in the primary dermatome and a lowered frequency of cutaneous dissemination. The interferon treated patients did not show a significant decrease in total healing time but they did have significant amelioration of post-herpetic neuralgia. Some toxicity was encountered in this trial in the form of fever, malaise, myalgia, and depressed leukocyte counts. The usefulness of leukocyte interferon for treatment of herpes zoster infections in the immunocompromised host will likely be expanded with the availability of recombinant DNA produced interferon. With the availability of large quantities of inexpensive and pure interfersons, these studies will be repeated with larger numbers of patients.

Acyclovir has been shown useful in a large controlled study for decreasing complications of cutaneous dissemination and visceral disease when data are combined for these two events[50,51]. This latter drug is of particular interest in that it has been demonstrated to have a good therapeutic index for the management of primary genital herpes simplex virus infections and hepes simplex virus infections in the immunocompromised host. Transfer factor has been considered for therapy but is not being rigorously evaluated[49].

CYTOMEGALOVIRUS INFECTION

Clinical Background. Human cytomegaloviruses are among the most ubiquitous of organisms capable of infecting humans. These viruses produce a broad spectrum of clinical disease ranging from asymptomatic or symptomatic infections in the newborn to life-threatening diseases in the immunocompromised host. World-wide, human cytomegaloviruses cause congenital infection in approximately 0.5-2.0 percent in all live births[52-54]. Although the majority of these children are born completely without symptoms, upwards of 5-15 percent will ultimately develop significant hearing, developmental, and/or visual impairment. Furthermore, 5-10 percent of children, depending upon circumstances, will acquire cytomegalovirus infection in the period immediately surrounding birth by contact with infected genital secretions, through ingestion of infected breast milk or via blood products[55-57]. The consequences of these infections are less apparent although it has been learned that pneumonia in the young infant, acute perinatal morbidity and mononucleosis syndromes in later infancy can result from these kinds of infections[58,59]. Cytomegalovirus infections in adults are most frequently asymptomatic; however, in the presence of immunosuppression, infection can be of clinical significance. Individuals receiving organ transplants including renal, bone marrow, and cardiac transplant recipients are all at risk for severe and even life-threatening cytomegalovirus infections, particularly pneumonitis[60,61]. It has been reported that the mortality of cytomegalovirus pneumonia in bone marrow transplant recipients alone ranges between 45-90 percent. Furthermore, cytomegalovirus has been associated with development of acquired immunodeficiency syndrome and Kaposi's sarcoma[62].

Under the conditions of organ transplantation, virtually every patient will develop cytomegalovirus infection. These data have been recently reviewed by Ho[63]. In a series of fifteen studies which included over 1,100 renal transplant recipients, the incidence of excretion of cytomegalovirus was 71 percent. Primary infection occurred in 53 percent of patients while reactivation occurred in 85 percent of individuals. In several of the studies the rate of reactivation was between 90-100 percent. The factors which influence the expression of infection post-transplantation include the underlying disease, the type of medication administered (cytotoxic or cytolytic), and host or graft rejection. Virus can be obtained from the environment, nosocomial contact from transfusion of blood, particularly, white cells and from the graft itself.

Regarding primary infection, there is strong epidemiologic evidence to suggest that the donated kidney is the primary source of cytomegalovirus infection. In this situation the seronegative organ transplant recipient would receive a kidney from a seropositive donor; however, the search for cytomegalovirus in the donor kidney has often been futile. The epidemiologic evidence suggesting that the kidney is a source of infection comes from the prospective studies of Ho[64] and Betts[65]. In these studies seronegative recipients that received kidneys from seropositive donors had infection rates of nearly 80 percent. While those who received kidneys from seronegative donors had infection rates of only 30 percent.

The situation is somewhat different in the case of bone marrow transplantation. It has been recognized by several investigators that the donor serologic status had no effect on subsequent morbidity and mortality caused by cytomegalovirus infection, as the incidence of cytomegalovirus infection in recipients of seropositive marrows was 35 percent whereas 52 percent of marrow recipients whose donors were seronegative became infected[66]. These factors were also examined by Myers and colleagues[67], in which the rate of infection in seronegative and seropositive recipients were similar for all groups varying between 53 and 64 percent with an overall average of 58 percent.

Clinical manifestations of cytomegalovirus infections in these patient populations can be particularly perplexing. As shown in Figure 3, primary and reactivated infections occur

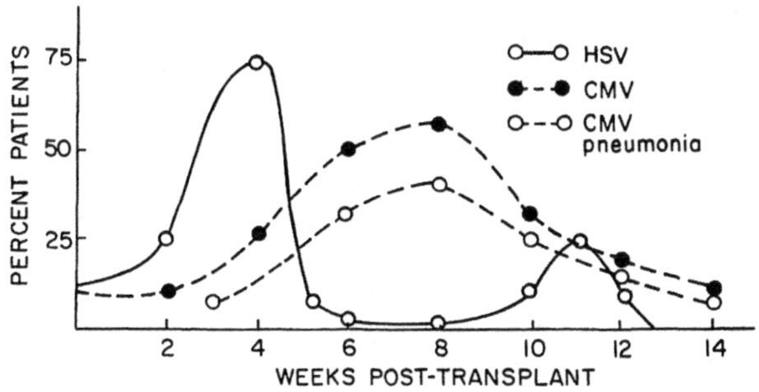

Fig. 3. Cytomegalovirus infection in patients with bone marrow transplantation.

approximately two to three months after transplantation with a range of one to four months. Not infrequently cytomegalovirus infection, even in the immunosuppressed patient can be asymptomatic. When symptomatic, febrile mononucleosis syndrome appears to be the most common presentation with the hallmark being prolonged fever and mild hepatitis[68]. With primary infection in over two-thirds of patients appear to have viremia and closer to 90 percent have viruria.

The next most common symptomatic manifestation of cytomegalovirus infection is pneumonitis, a complication which is particularly troublesome. The course of cytomegalovirus pneumonia varies strikingly from complete recovery to death. In renal transplant recipients mortality has been reported to be approximately 50 percent[68].

Other complications of significance in these patients are hepatitis and retinitis of varying severity. Hepatitis is not usually a serious problem following renal transplantation while cytomegalovirus retinitis is associated with significant visual impairment.

DIAGNOSIS

As with the other herpesviruses, isolation of cytomegalovirus in tissue culture remains the standard for diagnosis. However, in contrast to other herpesviruses the serologic diagnosis although useful may require so much time that it is often retrospective in nature. Virus may be recovered from body fluids or from tissues obtained from either biopsy or at autopsy. Cytomegaloviruses can be isolated from urine, blood, throat washings, saliva, tears, milk, semen, stool, and vaginal or cervical secretions. Biologic specimens can be inoculated directly into susceptible cell lines. Such lines include: human fibroblasts, either developed in one's own laboratory or obtained commercially. Commercial strains include WI38 or MA184 human embryonic fibroblasts. Cultures inoculated with virus containing material may show cytopathic effect in three to four days but generally between two and three weeks. Enlarged, rounded refactile cells appear in the center of the cell sheet rather than on the periphery of the monolayer. The cytopathic effect follows a linear pattern such that viral replication eventually destroy the entire monolayer.

Alternative methods of diagnosis include examination of urinary sediment by hematoxylin and eosin or Giemsa stains in order to demonstrate evidence of cytoplasmic inclusions. Electron microscopy can also be useful for these purposes.

A variety of serologic studies have been developed to

determine the prevalance of antibodies to cytomegalovirus infections both for diagnostic and for sero-epidemiologic studies. As with the other herpesviruses, these antibody studies include complement fixation, neutralization, fluorescence antibody, membrane antigens, enzyme linked immunosorbent assays, and immune adherence hemagglutination assays, among others. These assays have all been reviewed in detail[63,69].

TREATMENT

With the advent of organ transplantation, particularly renal allograft, heart, and bone marrow, and the requisite immunosuppressive therapy to maintain the transplanted graft, a high incidence of herpesvirus infections has been noted post-transplantation. This is particularly true for cytomegalovirus infections, both primary and recurrent. Of particular concern is the high mortality rate associated with cytomegalovirus pneumonia in the bone marrow transplant recipients. Thus, even with successful transplantation, the viral complication may be of such severity as to lead to early demise or loss of the transplanted organ.

Because of the high mortality in these patient populations, interferon and nucleoside analogs have been used alone and in combination. Meyers and colleagues have attempted to establish successful therapeutics for biopsy proven cytomegalovirus pneumonia but to no avail. Human leucocyte interferon at dosages of .2-6.4 X 10^5 units/kg/day administered at the time of diagnosis failed to alter the clinical expression of cytomegalovirus pneumonia in these patient populations[70]. similarly, vidarabine and acyclovir alone or administered with interferon were also of no value[71]. Importantly, the lung biopsies from these patients contained large quantities of virus. Thus, as a therapeutic for existing disease, interferon, vidarabine, and acyclovir do not appear to be useful.

Renal transplant recipients often suffer from cytomegalovirus infections. Beginning initially with vidarabine administration, Chien and colleagues were able to demonstrate that vidarabine therapy decreased viruria coincident of administration of study medication. Nevertheless, in many of these patients virus was persistently found in organs at autopsy[72]. Similar studies by Rytel drew analogous conclusions[73]. Vidarabine is ineffective in eliminating cytomegalovirus from the immunosuppressed host and, at best, has a transient effect on decreasing the quantity of virus excreted in the urine but without clinical benefit. Marker noted significant neurotoxicity with administration of this drug in patients with poor renal function[74].

In the heart transplant patient, cytomegalovirus retinitis is a grave consequence in a few patients. Pollard and colleagues have successfully shown that high-dose vidarabine is helpful in the prevention of this progressive disease[75].

More recently, a controlled study has been reported in the immunocompromised host principally suffering from cytomegalovirus viremia, utilizing the drug acyclovir[76]. This compound is most useful for herpes simplex infections.

The controlled studies of Balfour suggested an earlier time to defervescence and resolution of clinical symptomatology in patients receiving 1500 mg/m^2 of acyclovir intravenously[76]. These studies are being further assessed in an ongoing trial.

CONCLUSION

Herpesvirus infections of the immunocompromised host are exceedingly common with the increasing regimens for immunosuppression in individuals suffering from malignancy and the increasing frequency of organ transplantation. It is extremely likely that the frequency of these infections and the need for developing therapeutic approaches will remain popular in the medical community. To date, we have seen advances in the development of antiviral agents for the control of these infections, yet, it will be important to further develop means by which these infections can be prevented in the immunocompromised host. The development of acyclovir is a step in the direction of treatment of severe herpesvirus in these patient populations. Clearly, further therapeutic avenues need to evolve for the management of cytomegalovirus infections in organ transplant recipients as they remain a significant cause of mortality and morbidity.

ACKNOWLEDGEMENTS

Studies performed by the author and reported in this manuscript were supported in part by research grants from the National Institute of Allergy and Infectious Diseases (N01-AI-12667), by grants from the National Cancer Institute (CA-13148), and (RR-032) from the General Clinical Research Centers Programs, National Institutes of Health, and by the Robert Meyer Foundation.

REFERENCES

1. Levine, A.S., Schmipff, S.C., Graw, R., Jr., et al., Hematologic malignancies and other marrow failure stats: Progress in the management of complicating infections, Semin. Hematol., 11:141 (1974).
2. Pass, R.F., Whitley, R.J., Whelchel, J.D., Diethelm, A.G., Reynolds, D.W., Alford, C.A., Identification of patients with increased risk of infection with herpes simplex virus after renal transplantation, J. Infect. Dis. 140:487-492 (1979).
3. Korsager, B., Spencer, E.S., Mordhorst, C.J., Andersen, H.K., Herpesvirus hominis infections in renal transplant recipients, Scand. J. Infect. Dis. 7:11-19 (1975).
4. Montgomerie, J.Z., Becroft, D.M.O., Croxson, M.C., Doak, P.B., North, J.D.K., Herpes simplex virus infection after renal transplantation, Lancet 11:867-871 (1969)
5. Naraqi, S., Jackson, G.G., Jonasson, O.M., Yamashiroy, H.M., Prospective study of prevalence, incidence, and source of herpesvirus infections in patients with renal allografts, J. Infect. Dis. 136:531-540 (1977).
6. Meyers, J.D., Flournoy, N., Thomas, E.d., Infection with herpes simplex virus and cell-mediated immunity after marrow transplant, J. Infect. Dis. 142:336-346 (1980).
7. Spruance, S.L., Overall, J.C., Jr., Kern, E.R., Krueger, G.G., Pliam, V., Miller, W., The natural history of recurrent herpes simplex labialis. Implications for antiviral therapy, N. Engl. J. Med. 297:69-75 (1977).
8. Whitley, R.J., Levin, M., Barton, R., Hershey, B.J., Dvis, G., Keeney, R.W., Welchel, J., Diethelm, A.G., Kartus, P., and Soong, S.J., Herpes simplex virus infections in the immunocompromised host: natural history and topical acyclovir therapy, J. Infect. Dis. In Press (1983).
9. Muller, S.A., Herrmann, E.D., Jr., Winkelmann, R.K., Herpes simplex virus infections in hematoligic malignancies, Am. J. Med. 52:102-114 (1972).
10. Herout, V., Vortel, V., Vondrackova, A., Herpes simplex involvement of the lower respiratory tract, Am. J. Clin. Path. 46:411-419 (1966).
11. Linnemann, C.C., Jr., First, M.R., Alvira, M.M., Alexander, J.W., Schiff, G.M., Herpesvirus hominis type 2 meningoencephalitis following renal transplantation, Am. J. Med. 61:703-708 (1976).
12. Meyers, J.D., Flournoy, N., Thomas, E.D., Infection with herpes simplex virus and cell-mediated immunity after marow transplant, J. Infect. Dis. 142:338-346 (1980).
13. Lam, M.T., Pazin, G.J., Armstrong, J.A., Ho, M., Herpes simplex infection in acute myelogenous leukemia and other hematologic malignancies: a prospective study, Cancer 48:2168-2171 (1981).

14. Rawls, W.E., Herpes simplex viruses types 1 & 2 and herpesvirus simae, in Diagnostic Procedures for Viral, Richettsial and Chlamydial Infections, Editors: F. H. Lennette and N.J. Schmedt, American Public Health Association, New York, pp. 309-374 (1979).
15. Meyers, J.D., Wade, J.C., Mitchell, C.D., Saral, R., Lietman, P.S., Durack, D.T., Levin, M.J., Segreti, A.C., Balfour, H.H., Multicenter collaborative trial of intravenous acyclovir for tretment of mucocutaneous herpes simplex virus infection in the immunocompromised host, Am. J. Med. 73:229-236 (1982).
16. Saral, R., Burns, W.H., Laskin, O.L., et al., Acyclovir prophylaxis of herpes simplex virus infection, N. Engl. J. Med. 305:63-67 (1982).
17. Wade, J.C., Newton, B., McLaren, C., et al., Intravenous acyclovir to treat mucocutaneous herpes simplex virus infection after marrow transplantation, Ann. Intern. Med. 96:265-269 (1982).
18. Whitley, R.J., Soong, S.J., Dolin, R., Galasso, G.J., Chien, L.T., Alford, C.A., and the Collaborative Antiviral Study Group, Adenine arabinoside therapy of biopsy-proved herpes simplex encephalitis: National Institute of Allergy and Infectious Diseases Collaborative Antiviral Study, N. Engl. J. Med. 297:289-294 (1977).
19. Whitley, R.J., Soong, S.J., Hirsch M.S., Karchmer, A.W., Dolin, R., Galasso, G., Dunnick, J.K., Alford, C.A., Jr. and the NIAID Collaborative Antiviral Study Group: Herpes simplex encephalitis: vidarabine therapy and diagnostic problems, N. Engl. J. Med. 304:313-318 (1981).
20. Whitley, R.J., Hilty, M., Haynes, R., Bryson, Y., Connor, J.D., Soong, S.J., Alford, C.A., Jr., and the NIAID Collaborative Antiviral Study Group: Herpes simplex encephalitis: vidarabine therapy of varicella in immunosuppressed patients, J. Pediat. 101:125-131 (1982).
21. Whitley, R.J., Yeager, A., Kartus, P., Bryson, Y., Connor, J.D., Aahmias, A.J., Soong, S.J., and the NIAID Collaborative Antiviral Study Group, Neonatal herpes simplex virus infection: follow-up evaluation of vidarabine therapy, (In Press), Pediatrics
22. Whitley, R.J., Spruance, S., Hayden, F.G., Overall, J., Alford, C.A., Gwaltney, J.M., Soong, S.J., and the NIAID Collaborative Antiviral Study Group: Vidarabine therapy of mucocutaneous herpes simplex virus infections in the immunocompromised host, J. Infect. Dis. (In Press).
23. Feldman, S., Hughes, W.T., and Daniel, G.B., Varicella in children with cancer: seventy-seven cases, Pediatrics 56:388 (1975).
24. Falliers, D.J., and Ellis, E.F., Corticosteroids and varicella: six year experience in an asthmatic population, Arch. Dis. Child. 40:593 (1965).

25. Whitley, R.J., Hilty, M., Haynes, R., Bryson, Y., Connor, J.D., Soong, S.J., Alford, C.A., Jr., and NIAID Collaborative Antiviral Study Group, Vidarabine therapy of varicella in immunosuppressed patients, J. Pediat. 1:125 (1982).
26. Arvin, A.M., Kushner, J.H., Feldman, S., Buchner, R.L. , Hammond, D., Merigan, T.C., Human leukocyte interferon for treatment of varicella in children with cancer, N. Engl. J. Med. 306:761 (1982).
27. Whitley, R.J., Soong, S.J., Dolin, R., Betts, R., Linnemann, C., Jr., Alford, C.A., Jr., and the NIAID Collaborative Antiviral Study Group, Early vidarabine therapy to control the complications of herpes zoster in immunosuppressed patients, N. Engl. J. Med. 307:971 (1982).
28. Wller, T.H., Varicella-zoster virus, in Diagnostic Procedures for Viral, Richettsial and Chlamydial Infections, Editors: F.H. Lennette and N.J. Schmedt, American Public Health Association, New York, pp. 375-398 (1979).
29. Ross, A.H., Modification of chickenpox in family contacts by administration of gamma globulin, N. Engl. J. Med. 267:369 (1962).
30. Brunell, P.A., Ross, A., Miler, L., and Kuo, B, Prevention of varicella by zoster immune globulin, N. Engl. J. Med. 280:1191 (1969).
31. Brunell, P.A., Gershon, A.A., Hughes, W.T., Riley, H.D., and Smith, J., Prevention of varicella in high-risk children: a collaborative study, Pediatrics 50:718 (1972).
32. Brunell, P.A., and Grshon, A.A., Passive immunization against varicella-zoster infections and other modes of therapy, J. Infect. Dis. 127:415 (1973).
33. Report of the Comittee on Infectious Diseases, American Academy of Pediatrics, 18th Edition, P. 285 (1982).
34. Takahashi, M., Okuno, Y., Otsuka, T., Osame, J. Takamizawa, A., Sasada, T., and Kubo, T., Development of a liver attenuated varicella vaccine, Biken J. 18:25 (1975).
35. Takahashi, M., Otsuka, T., Okuno, Y., Asano, Y., Yazaki, T., Isomura, S., Live vaccine used to prevent the spread of varicella in children in hospital, Lancet 2:1288 (1974).
36. Izawa, T., Ihara, T., Hattori, A., Iwasa, T., Kamiya, H., Sakurai, M., and TAkahashi, M., Application of a live varicella vaccine in children with acute leukemia or other malignant diseases, Pediatrics 60:805 (1977).
37. Asano, Y., Nakayama, H., Yazaki, T., Kato, R., Hirose, S., Tsuzuki, K., Ito, S., Isomura, S., and TAkahashi, M., Protection against varicella in family contacts by immediate inoculation with live varicella vaccine, Pediatrics 59:3 (1977).

38. Ha, K., Baba, K., Ikeda, T., Nishida, M., Yabuuchi, H., and Takahashi, M., Application of live varicella vaccine to children with acute leukemia or other malignancies without suspension of anticancer therpy, Pediatrics 65:346 (1980).
39. Barrett, F.F., Wexler, M.L., and Douglas, R.G., Treatment of progressive varicella with cytarabine, Tex. Med. 68:65 (1972).
40. Chow, A.W., Forester, J.H., Ryniuk, W., Cytosine arabinoside therapy for herpesvirus infections, Antimicrob Agents Chemother. 1970:214 (1971).
41. Hall, T.C., Wilfert, C., Jaffe, N., Traggis, D., Lux, S., RAmpf, P., and Kate, S., Treatment of varicella-zoster with cytosine arabinoside, Trans. Assoc. Am. Phys. 82:201 (1969).
42. Prager, D., Bruder, M., Sawitsky, A., Disseminated varicella in a patient with acute myelogenous leukemia: treatment with cytosine arabinoside, J. Pediat. 81:562 (1972).
44. Cowdry, E.V., The problem of intranuclear inclusions in virus diseases, Arch. Pathol. 18:527 (1934).
45. Stevens, D.A., and Merigan, T.C., Interferon, antibody, and other host factors, in herpes zoster, J. Clin. Invest. 51:1170 (1972).
46. Eaglstein, W.H., Katz, R., and Brown, J.A., The effects of early corticosteroid therapy on the skin eruption and pain of herpes zoster, J.A.M.A. 211:1681 (1970).
47. Whitley, R.J., Soong, S.J., Dolin, R., Betts, R., Linnemann, C., Jr., Alford, C.A., Jr., and the NIAID Collaborative Antiviral Study Group, Early vidarabine therapy to control the complications of herpes zoster in immunosupressed patients, N. Engl. J. Med. 307:971 (1982).
48. Merigan, T.C., Rand, K.H., and Pollard, R.B., Human leukocyte interferon for the treatment of herpes zoster in patients with cancer, N. Engl. J. Med. 298:981 (1978).
49. Steele, R.W., Myers, M.G., and Vincent, M.M., Transfer factor for the pevention of varicella-zoster infection in childhood leukemia, N. Engl. J. Med. 303:355 (1980).
50. Essman, V. Ipsen, J, Peterslund, N.A., Seyer-Hansen, K., Schonheyder, H., Henning, J., Therapy of acute herpes zoster with acyclovir in the nonimmunocompromised host, Am. J. Med. 73:320 (1982).
51. Balfour, H.H., Bean, B., Laskin, O.L., et. al., Acyclovir halts progression of herpes zoster in immunocompromised patients, N. Engl. J. Med. 308:1448-1453 (1983).
52. Henshaw, J. B., Scheiner, A.P., Moxley, A.W., et al., School failure and deafness after "silent" cytomegalovirus infections, N. Engl. J. Med. 295:468 (1976).

53. Stagno, S., Reynolds, D.W., Tsiantos, A., et. al., Comparative serial virologic and serologic studies of symptomatic and subclinical congenitally and natally acquire cytomegalovirus infections, J. Infect. Dis. 132:568 (1975).
54. Lang, D.J., The epidemiology of cytomegalovirus infections: interpretation of recent observations, in Infections of the Fetus and the Newborn Infant, Krugman, S., and Gershon, A.A., (eds.), Alan R. Liss (New York), pp. 35-45 (1975).
55. Stagno, S., Reynolds, D.W., Pass, R.F., et. al., Breast milk and the risk of cytomegalovirus infection, N. Engl. J. Med. 302:1073-1076 (1980).
56. Reynolds, D.W., Stagno, S., Hosty, T.S., Tiller, M., and Alford, C.A., Jr., Maternal cytomegalovirus excretion and perinatal infections, N. Engl. J. Med. 289:1-5 (1973).
57. Yeager, A.S., Transfusion acquired cytomegalovirus infection in newborn infants, Am. J. Dis. Child. 128:478-483 (1974).
58. Stagno, S., Brasfield, D.M., Brown, M.B., Cassell, G.H., Pifer, L.L., Whitley, R.J., and Tiller, R.E., Infant pneumonitis associated with cytomegalovirus, chlamydia, pneumocystis, and ureaplasma: a prospective study, Pediatrics 68:322-329 (1981).
59. Yeager, A.S. and Palumbo, P.E., Symptomatic cytomegalovirus infection in premature infants following transmission of virus from mother to infant. (Presented at the Conference on Pathogenesis and Prevention of Human Cytomegalovirus Infection: Philadelphia, Pennsylvania: April 20-22) (1983).
60. Rubin, R.J., Russell, P.S., Levin, M., et. al., Summary of a workshop on cytomegalovirus infections during organ transplantation, J. Infect. Dis.139:728-734 (1979).
61. Meyers, J.D., Spencer, H.C., Jr., Watts, J.C., et. al., Cytomegalovirus pneumonia after human marrow transplantation, Ann. Intern. Med. 82:181-182 (1975).
62. Drew, W.L., Mintz, L., Miner, R.C., Sans, M., and Ketterer, D., Prevalence of cytomegalovirus infection in homosexual men, J. Infect. Dis. 143:188-192 (1981).
63. Ho, M., Human cytomegalovirus infections in immunosuppressed patients, in Cytomegalovirus: Biology and Infection, Greenough, W.B. and Merigan, T.C. (eds), Plenum (New York), pp. 171-204 (1982).
64. Ho, M. Suwansirikul, S., Dowling, J.N., Youngblood, L.A., Armstrong, J.A., The transplanted kidney as a source of cytomegalovirus infections, N. Engl. J. Med. 293:1109-1112 (1975).
65. Betts, R.F., Freeman, R.B., Douglas, R.G., Jr., Talley, T.E., Rundell, B., Transmission of cytomegalovirus infection with renal allograft, Kidney Int. 8:387-394 (1975).

66. Neiman, P.E., Reeves, W., Ray, G., Flournoy, N., Lerner, K.G., Sale, G.E., Thomas, E.D., A prospective analysis of interstitial pneumonia and opportunistic viral infection among recipients of allogenic bone marrow grafts, J. Infect. Dis. 136:754-767 (1977).
67. Meyers, J.D., Spencer, H.C., Jr., Watts, J.C., Gregg, M.B., Stewart, J.A., Troupin, R.H., Thomas, E.D., Cytomegalovirus pneumonia after human marrow transplantation, Ann. Intern. Med. 82:181-188 (1975).
68. Rubin, R.H., Cosimi, A.B., Tolkoff-Rubin, N.E., Russell, P.S., Hirsch, M.D., Infectious disease syndromes attributable to cytomegalovirus and their significance among renal transplant recipients, Transplantation 24:458-464 (1977).
69. Reynolds, D.W., Stagno, S., Alford, C.A., Jr., Laboratory diagnosis of cytomegalovirus infections, in Diagnostic Procedures for Viral, Richettsial and Chlamydial Infections, Editors: F.H. Lennette and N.J. Schmedt, American Public Health Association, New York, p. 399-439 (1979).
70. Meyers, J.D., McGuffin, R.W., Neiman, P.E., et. al., Toxicity and efficacy of human leukocyte interferon for treatment of cytomegalovirus pneumonia after marrow transplantation, J. Infect. Dis. 141:555-562 (1980).
71. Meyers, J.D., CMV infection after bone marrow transplantation, Conference on Pathogenesis and Prevention of Human Cytomegalovirus Infection, Philadelphia, Pennsylvania, April 20-22 (1983).
72. Chein, L.T., Cannon, M.J., Whitley, R.J., et. al., Effect of adenine arabinoside on cytomegalovirus infections, J. Infect. Dis. 130:32-39 (1974).
73. Rytel, M.W. and Kauffman, H.M., Clinical efficacy of adenin e arabinoside in therapy of cytomegalovirus infections in renal allograft recipients, J. Infect. Dis. 133:202-205 (1976).
74. Marker, S.G., Howard, R.J., Groth, K.E., et. al., A trial of vidarabine for cytomegalovirus infection in renal transplant patients, Arch. Intern. Med. 140-1441-1444 (1980).
75. Pollard, R.B., Egbert, P.R., Gallagher, J.G., et. al., Cytomegalovirus retinitis in immunosuppressed hosts, I. Natural history and effects of treatment with adenine arabinoside, Ann. Intern. Med. 93:655-660 (1980).
76. Balfour, H.H., Jr., Bean, B., Mitchell, C.D., Sachs, G.W., Boen, J.R., Kedelman, C.K., Acyclovir in immunocompromised patients with cytomegalovirus disease. A controlled trial at one institution, Am. J. Med. 73:241-248 (1982).

FUNGAL INFECTIONS IN THE COMPROMISED HOST - AN OVERVIEW

Richard D. Diamond

Associate Professor of Medicine and Microbiology
Boston University School of Medicine
Boston, Massachusetts

INTRODUCTION

For those interested in medical mycology, the 1960s and 70s represented a period dedicated to raising the awareness of others to the clinical importance of opportunistic mycoses. The medical literature of that period is replete with examples dedicated to this goal, as clinicians who dealt regularly with immunocompromised patients became increasingly aware of the scope of the problem. For example, Hart et al emphasized that most mycoses observed in normal hosts were caused by a characteristic group of fungi, including coccidioidomycosis, histoplasmosis, cryptococcosis, mycetoma, blastomycosis and sporotrichosis; in contrast, compromised patients tended to develop candidiasis, aspergillosis and mucormycosis, as well as disseminated forms of cryptococcosis, histoplasmosis, and coccidioidomycosis[1]. Thus, it became clear that as prolonging the survival of immuno- compromised patients became more feasible, increasing numbers of these patients were developing infections, such as disseminated candidiasis, aspergillosis and mucormycosis, rarely seen in normal hosts. Moreover, when infected with fungi which usually cause self-limited disease in normal hosts, those with abnormal host defenses more often developed progressive, disseminated mycoses. Other investigators reporting series of patients collected both from results of postmortem or clinical series noted systemic fungal infections in 10-58% of cases of hematologic malignancies[1-6]. When time periods were compared, the frequency of such mycoses was observed to have increased 2- to 4-fold or more[6-8]. In such series, generally candidiasis was most common, followed by aspergillosis (ahead of candidiasis in some series), then cryptocococcosis and mucormycosis. Similarly, renal allograft (and, more recently, bone marrow transplant) recipients developed mycoses in 13-45% of cases in different reported series[9-11]. Clearly, systemic mycoses were recognized as an emerging factor of great import to the survival of immunocompromised patients.

DEFINITIONS

Because definitions used in different reports may vary, it is necessary to specify criteria which separate systemic mycoses from the local infections which also occur in patients with severe impairment of host defenses, but may occur in less compromised or even apparently normal patients as well. Systemic candidiasis, then, refers to invasion of tissues beyond mucocutaneous surface structures, e.g., skin and its appendages (hair and nails), oral cavity, vagina, etc. In contrast to Candida, local tissue-invasive lesions are not caused by Aspergillus or the fungi causing mucormycosis in the absence of significant host defense defects; therefore, systemic aspergillosis refers to hyphal invasion of host tissues at any site. This is distinct from cases where hyphae are present within sinuses, bronchi or well-encapsulated cavitary pulmonary lesions without penetration into surrounding tissues.

HOST DEFENSE FACTORS

The specific type of underlying deficit in host defense mechanism determines which fungi are likely to act as opportunistic in any given patient. Immunocompromise takes many forms. However, in the U.S.A. at this time, the largest body of objective data comes from the group of patients accounting for most opportunistic mycoses: those with neutropenia or receiving therapy with cytotoxic agents or corticosteroid therapy. This includes patients with hematologic malignancies as well as those undergoing immunosuppression to prevent transplant rejection. Of course, numerous other factors may compromise host defenses and predispose to mycotic infections in other groups of patients, or add to the host defense deficits present in neutropenic patients and those receiving corticosteroids and cytotoxic drugs. These include genetic disorders, diabetes mellitus, malnutrition, and extensive trauma, including burns among others.

In some cases, it is possible to associate the apparent predisposing factors in individual patients with specific mycoses which are more likely to occur. For example, systemic candidiasis appears to occur most often in two distinct groups: neutropenic patients and patients who have had extensive surgery (or trauma), accompanied by malnutrition (often requiring intravenous hyperalimentation) and prolonged courses of broad-spectrum antibacterial chemotherapy. Similarly, patients with neutropenia are at risk for invasive aspergillosis. Where hereditary disorders of neutrophil function are present, as in chronic granulomatous disease, systemic aspergillosis (or candidiasis) is a common complication[12]. Systemic aspergillosis also may occur in non-neutropenic patients receiving corticosteroids and/or chemotherapy with cytotoxic agents. When associated with neoplasms rather than with diabetic ketoacidosis alone, mucormycosis tends to occur in leukopenic patients with leukemias or lymphoma patients who also have diabetes mellitus[13]. Other systemic mycoses are more likely to be present even in the absence of neutropenia, where compromise in host cell-mediated immune mechanisms predominates. Thus, cryptococcosis is likely to be seen in patients with Hodgkin's disease, other lymphomas or lymphoreticular malignancies, as well as in those receiving corticosteroid therapy[14]. Patients with the acquired immunodeficiency syndrome (AIDS) are at risk for a wide array of infections by virtue of a broad deficit in cell-mediated immune function. Cryptococcosis, as would be expected, is among this group of infections. In contrast, while mucocutaneous candidiasis commonly causes significant problems, systemic candidiasis is a rare complication in AIDS patients (as is systemic aspergillosis). Patients with cell-mediated immune defects also are at increased risk for reactivation or progressive dissemination of primary coccioidomycosis or histoplasmosis. In many cases, however, it is impossible in individual patients to make a clear judgment as to which mycoses are most likely because multiple deficits in host defense mechanisms coexist. For example, prolonged neutropenia often occurs in patients with lymphomas by virtue of treatment with cytotoxic chemotherapy. Such a severely immunocompromised host is at risk for rapidly progressive infections caused by a broad array of organisms.

CLINICAL FEATURES AFFECTING DIAGNOSIS

Early diagnosis of opportunistic mycoses is, at once, extremely difficult yet critically important. In the cases of neutropenic patients with mycoses, most of the early series were based upon data obtained at postmortem. Few of these infections were diagnosed during life, and fewer were sucessfully treated. However, at least some cases diagnosed early in the course of these mycoses can be treated successfully[15]. Even in the case of cryptococcosis, usually a more chronic infection where cell-mediated immune deficits predominate rather than neutropenia, the presence of preexisting immunocompromise reduces the likelihood of permanent cure[14].

Thus, careful and thorough clinical evaluation of patients at high risk for systemic fungal infections is of paramount importance. The history should include a thorough review of exposure to immunocompromising drugs as well as presence of disease states which predispose to mycoses. In addition, recent or remote residence in endemic areas for histoplasmosis and coccidioidomycosis should be documented. General findings, such as fever and malaise, are often less prominent than in bacterial infections, especially in cryptococcosis and mucormycosis.

In candidiasis, mucocutaneous lesions may cause significant morbidity by themselves, and may provide a source of organisms for systemic infections in susceptible patients where portals of entry exist (e.g., intravenous catheters, ulcerations in the gastrointestinal tract). Soreness from extensive oral thrush or dysphagia secondary to esophagitis may impair food intake and thereby compromise nutrition in an already malnourished patient. Bladder wall invasion by Candida may be symptomatic as well. Systemic candidiasis may cause findings referable to the sites of specific lesions: arthritis, meningitis, perforation of an abdominal viscus, endocarditis (with or without embolization), loss of vision late in the course of endophthalmitis (a rare complication in leukopenic patients), colicky pain and tenderness arising from uretheral passages of fungus balls, nodular skin lesions on erythematous bases, and pneumonia (a late consequence of widespread, hematogenous dissemination). Other lesions in deep tissues such as the liver, spleen or kidneys may cause no apparent signs or symptoms.

Systemic aspergillosis almost always involves the lungs, though necrotic skin lesions, nasal or palatal necrosis, perforations of the gastrointestinal tract or focal neurologic findings secondary to cerebral infarction may predominate. Mucormycosis may cause lesions identical to those seen in aspergillosis, in addition to the necrotic lesions of the nose, palate, sinus, orbit and brain, which characteristically occur in association with diabetes ketoacidosis, but sometimes are observed in other patients as well.

Cryptococcosis most commonly causes signs and symptoms referable to the central nervous system, including papilledema, personality change, and cranial nerve palsies. Other than the latter, focal findings are unusual early in the course of cryptococcosis and prior to complicating seizures. Pulmonary lesions may be present. Though pulmonary lesions are usually focal and cause minimal symptoms, severely immunosuppressed patients, including those with AIDS, may have a diffuse pneumonia causing signs and symptoms of profound hypoxemia. Patients with disseminated cryptococcosis may also have focal lytic lesions in bones and skin lesions with a broad range of appearance.

Because of characteristic generalized involvement of the reticuloendothelial system, histoplasmosis should be suggested by signs thereof, such as hepatosplenomegaly, in addition to pulmonary lesions. Oral mucosal ulceration may be a useful sign as well. In contrast, coccidioidomycosis causes focal lesions in the lungs and elsewhere.

Given that all of the above findings are nonspecific, laboratory studies are crucial in the diagnosis of invasive mycoses. In some circumstances, laboratory findings make the diagnosis straightforward and relatively simple. For example, in cryptococcosis, positive tests for capsular polysaccharide antigen in serum or cerebrospinal fluid (especially in titers >1:8) or floridly positive smears should be confirmed by cultures, but this generally is easy to do in such circumstances. Likewise, bone marrow, blood buffy coat or biopsies of other organs of the reticuloendothelial system may be diagnostic in histoplasmosis. In general, observation of the pathogenic phase of a fungus (e.g., septate hyphae in aspergillosis, encapsulated yeasts in cryptococcosis, spherules in coccidioidomycosis) in material obtained from lesions is most useful in diagnosis. Thus, when positive, wet smears (with and without digestion with sodium or potassium hydroxide) and stained tissue specimens of such lesions can provide the most rapid diagnoses. Cultural confirmation may come later (or sometimes not at all). In addition, cultures must be interpreted carefully in aspergillosis and mucormycosis because spores of the causative organisms are common airborne contaminants of surfaces (including open culture plates). Thus, open skin lesions, nasal or palatal lesions of aspergillosis or mucormycosis are more reliably diagnosed by the characteristic appearance of hyphae on wet smears (though these mycoses cannot be ruled out if such smears are negative). Occasionally, smears of sputum will reveal hyphae in these diseases, especially if cavitation of pulmonary lesions has occurred. Sputum specimens from patients with a variety of lung diseases may culture _Aspergillus_ in the absence of tissue invasion by the fungus, and most patients who have been reported with invasive aspergillosis have had negative sputum cultures. However, in patients who are predisposed to aspergillosis by accompanying factors, a positive sputum culture cannot be ignored. When appropriate smears are negative, biopsy of documented lesions is the only completely reliable method for diagnosing aspergillosis or mucormycosis. Nevertheless, even open biopsies of lungs or other organs may reveal only nonspecific histological changes, such as hemorrhagic necrosis, and sections containing fungi may be missed. Diagnosis must then rely upon less specific criteria, including the status of the host, the setting and pulmonary infiltrate in relation to antibacterial therapy and rapid radiologic progression, often of a dense lesion or lesions which extend peripherally in lung fields and may cavitate. Blind biopsy of other organs outside the lung is rarely helpful, so is not indicated in diagnosis of these diseases.

In cryptococcosis, positive cultures of sputum, especially in patients with underlying lung disease but without hematologic malignancies, corticosteroid therapy or AIDS, are more likely to be indicative of saprophytic colonization than of tissue invasion. On chest x-rays, pulmonary cryptococcosis when apparent usually produces single or multiple mass lesions without cavitation or calcification; more diffuse, interstitial lesions may be present in severely immunocompromised patients. Definitive diagnosis of cryptococcosis requires isolation of the organism from cerebrospinal fluid, blood, urine or lesions in tissues.

Candidiasis presents an even greater diagnostic challenge. Wet smears showing characteristic combinations of yeasts and pseudohyphae are diagnostic of local tissue invasion, so can distinguish oral thrush or esophagitis from ulcers due to viruses, other infectious agents, or cytotoxic drugs. Esophageal candidiasis does not invariably produce abnormalities on barium swallow, nor are such abnormalities specific for candidiasis when observed. The presence of pseuodhyphae in fresh, clear urine specimens indicates the presence of invasive genitourinary candidiasis, though does not distinguish between local disease of the bladder wall mucosa and invasive, parenchymal renal lesions secondary to dissemination. Moreover, contamination of urine specimens with vaginal secretions may falsely suggest the presence of genitourinary candidiasis. Likewise, pseudohyphal forms seen in sputum may originate from oral or tracheobronchial mucosal lesions rather than invasive pulmonary candidiasis. The latter is generally a late complication of widespread hematogenous dissemination of candidiasis. Chest x-rays, if they are positive at all in this situation, show only diffuse, fine infiltration. Primary *Candida* pneumonia is extremely rare. In neutropenic patients, isolation of *Candida* from blood is likely to represent disseminated candidiasis[17], and this association is even more definite if no intravenous line is in place at the time of culture. However, the significance of candidemia is less certain in non-neutropenic patients. Moreover, from most series of disseminated candidiasis, at best only 25-40% of patients have positive blood cultures. Skin lesions may be present and focal lesions in other organs may yield organisms on biopsy.

More often than not, it is impossible to determine with absolute certainty whether or not systemic mycoses are present. Patients at highest risk for these infections often are thrombocytopenic, seriously increasing the risk of invasive diagnostic procedures usually required for definitive diagnosis. For this reason, it is critical to search for easily accessible lesions from which material can be obtained for diagnosis with minimal risk. Therefore, though not present in most systemic mycoses, any new skin lesion should be examined carefully in such patients.

Given the difficulties inherent in diagnosis of invasive mycoses, useful serologic procedures have been sought actively. While tests for cryptococcal antigen shave proven valuable, serologic tests for other mycoses remain experimental. Thus far, many procedures for detection of antibodies, antigens or both in body fluids have been shown to correlate with the presence of systemic candidiasis, and some promising result have been obtained in aspergillosis. However, results overlap between different groups of patients, so that no available test can distinguish between individual patients who need therapy and those who do not. Moreover, the experimental nature of these tests means that procedures are unstandardized between different laboratories and, even when available to clinicians, may not provide data on a timely enough basis to be of clinical utility, but rather merely prove to be of retrospective academic interest.

CURRENT TRENDS AND FUTURE PROSPECTS

Our increasing experience with systemic mycoses has many discouraging features. Diagnosis most often is uncertain and, even when disese is known to be present, available therapy has limited effectiveness and significant toxicity. However, the clinical importance of systemic mycoses now has been established firmly enough to permit investigators to stop discussing increasing disease incidences, and begin noting situations where progress has been made in decreasing the incidence of such infections. Thus, new protocols for prevention of graft rejection, including use of newer agents such as cyclosporin A, may decrease the risk of some opportunistic mycoses complicating transplantations. Likewise, a preliminary report suggests that patients with hematologic malignancies associated with persistent granulocytopenia and fever despite continuing antibacterial therapy benefit from empiric antifungal therapy[18]. It appears that, at least in some hospital settings where fungal superinfections are common, it may be possible to reduce the frequency of fatal systemic mycoses by preventing fungal superinfection and controlling clinically undetected fungal infections without unacceptable drug toxicity. In other settings, use of surveillance cultures has proven to be useful in better defining patients at risk for systemic candidiasis[19] or Trichosporon infections[20]. Additional studies will be required to determine whether or not such practices should become widely used. However, this type of positive result bodes well for a future where systemic mycoses will be more easily managed problems than they are now.

REFERENCES

1. Hart, P.D., Russel, E. Jr., and Remington, J.S, J.Infect. Dis. 120:169 (1969).
2. Chang, H., Rodriguez, V., Narboni, G., Bodey, G.P., Luna, M.A., and Freireich, E.J., Medicine (Baltimore) 55:259 (1976).
3. Singer, C., Kaplan, M.H., and Armstrong, D., Amer. J . Med. 62:731 (1977).
4. Mirsky, H., and Cuttner, J., Cancer 30:348 (1972).
5. DeGregorio, M.W., Les, W.M.F., Linker, C.A., Jacobs, R.A., and Ries, C.A., Amer. J. Med. 73:543 (1982)
6. Stahel, R.A., Vogt, P., Schuler, G., Ruttner, J.R., Frich, P., and Oelz, O., J. Infections 5:269 (1982).
7. Hotchi, M., Okada, MN., and Nasu, T., Amer. J. Clin. Pathol. 74:410 (1980).
8. Rose, H.D., and Varkey, B., Medicine (Baltimore) 54:499 (1975).
9. Bach, M.C., Adler, J.L., Breman, J., Fang-Ku, P., Sahyoun, A., Schlesinger, R.M., Madras, P., and Monaco, A.P., Lancet 1:180 (1973).
10. Rifkind, D., Marchroio, T.L., Sclmeck, S. A., and Hill, R.B., Amer. J. Med. 43:28 (1967).
11. Gallis, H.A., Berman, R.A., Cate, T.R., Hamilton, J.D., Gunnells, J.C., and Stickel, D.L., Arch. Intern. Med. 135:1163 (1975).
12. Cohen, M.S., Isturiz, R.E., Malech, H.L. et al,. Amer. J. Med. 71:59 (1981).
13. Meyer, R.D., Rosen, P., and Armstrong, D., Ann. Intern. Med. 77:871 (1972).
14. Diamond, R.D., and Bennett, J. E., Ann. Intern. Med. 80:176 (1974).
15. Pennington, J.E., N. Engl. J. Med. 295:426 (1976).
16. Young, R.C., Bennett, J.E., Geelhoed, G.W., and Levine, A.S., Ann. Intern. Med. 80:605 (1974).
17. Meunier-Carpentier, F., Kiehn, T.E., and Armstrong, D., Amer. J. Med. 71:363 (1981).
18. Pizzo, P.A., Robichard, K.J., Gill, F.A., and Witebsky, F.G., Amer. J. Med. 72:101 (1982).
19. Sandford, G.R., Merz, W.G., Wingard, J.R., Chrache, P., and Saral, R., J. Infect. Dis. 142:503 (1980).
20. Haupt, H.M., Merz, W.G., Beschorner, W.E., Vaughan, W.P., and Saral, R., J. Infect. Dis. 147:199 (1983).

SUSCEPTIBILITY TESTING OF MEDICALLY IMPORTANT FUNGI

William G. Merz

Department of Laboratory Medicine
The Johns Hopkins Medical Institutions
Baltimore, Maryland

INTRODUCTION

In vitro susceptibility testing can provide results to predict the antibiotic microorganism interactions which should correlate with *in vivo* efficacy. Generally, the results are expressed as the minimal inhibitory concentration (MIC), the lowest concentration of an agent which inhibits the growth of the microorganism, or as the minimal fungicidal concentration (MFC), the lowest concentration of an agent which kills a statistically significant number of organisms. These values are then correlated with attainable blood levels to determine whether the organism is susceptible or resistant. Finally, clinical correlation of efficacy and susceptibility or failure and resistance must be confirmed. Unfortunately, these principles have not been well established with fungal pathogens and antifungal agents. Interpretation of the *in vitro* susceptibility testing of antifungal agents suffers from the lack of standardized procedures. Variables, such as the type and size of the inoculum, the medium, temperature of incubation, length of incubation, and the definition end points must be standardized in order to compare susceptibility and efficacy results. A second problem is the paucity or lack of correlation of susceptibility data and clinical efficacy. Controlled studies and studies with appropriate animal models are needed to correlate the *in vitro* susceptibility data, blood levels of the antifungal agent, and clinical outcome for individual fungal infections.

Susceptibility testing of fungi has not been performed routinely in contrast to the susceptibility testing performed with bacterial pathogens. Amphotericin-B (Amp-B) has been the only systemic antifungal drug available until recently for the treatment of a wide spectrum of life-threatening fungal infections. Although clinical failures occur, especially with opportunistic fungi in the compromised host, testing of Amp-B has not routinely been performed due to lack of alternative drugs, the general predictability of susceptibility results with most species of human pathogenic fungi, and the lack of frequent development of resistance to Amp-B during therapy.

The need for fungal susceptibility testing may be indicated more today than in the past to provide clinicians with specific data to improve the management of life-threatening mycoses. The appropriate use of standardized, rapid, accurate susceptibility tests could:

1. Provide data on the newer antifungal drugs including the imidazoles, miconazole and ketoconazole, which may prove to be alternatives to Amp-B with certain clinical settings or mycoses.

2. Provide susceptibility data on fungi not previously associated with human infections, which are found causing opportunistic infections in compromised patients.

3. Detect the emergence of fungi resistant to antifungal drugs.

4. Provide data on the *in vitro* activity of combinations of antifungal drugs which may be synergistic.

5. Provide data to allow comparison of the *in vitro* antifungal activity of new compounds.

IN VITRO SUSCEPTIBILITY TESTING

In vitro susceptibility tests have been developed to assess the relative susceptibility of the medically important yeasts and filamentous fungi to amphotericin B, 5-fluorocytosine, and the imidazoles, miconazole and ketoconazole. In general, interpretation of the significance of susceptibility data suffers from the lack of clinical data correlating the *in vitro* susceptibility tests with treatment successes or failures as well as the lack of standardized testing to insure comparable results among laboratories.

Amphotericin-B

Susceptibility testing of fungi to Amp-B is not routinely conducted, in spite of the fact that it is the most commonly administered antifungal drug, and in spite of the fact that failures or relapses are not uncommon. Broth dilution (macro and micro), disk diffusion, semi-solid agar, agar dilution[1] and radiometric techniques[2] have been developed for Amp-B susceptibility testing. Due to the insolubility of Amp-B (or other polyene antifungals) and to its decomposition due to temperature, susceptibility tests must be controlled to insure the validity of the results.

Most medically important fungi (yeasts, agents of systemic mycoses, some Aspergillus isolates, and most zygomycetes) are susceptibile to Amp-B[1]. Fungi commonly resistant de novo to Amp-B include some isolates of Aspergillus, Pseudallescheria boydii, and certain species of dematiaceous fungi. Most relapses or treatment failures are probably not due to the development of Amp-B resistant fungi. Examples of the development of resistance during therapy do occur, but the frequency is unknown. Isolates of Aspergillus spp. have been shown to have progressively increasing MIC's to Amp-B during therapy. In addition, more recent reports document the recovery of resistant isolates of yeasts with MIC $\geq$ 2 - > 100 µg/ml). The recovery of resistant isolates of C. albicans[3], C. tropicalis[4,5], C. parapsilosis[5], and C. neoformans[9] from clinical specimens raises the question of the frequency and significance of this occurence. The mechanism of resistance has usually been associated with the loss of ergosterol, the binding site for Amp-B in the cell membrane[10]. the majority of the resistant yeast isolates were recovered from immunocompromised patients receiving cytoxic drugs (possibly mutagens), antibacterial antibiotics suppressing normal bacterial competition, and long courses or oral non-absorbable or systemic polyene therapies. These conditions may provide an environment for the emergence of progressively more resistant populations of Amp-B resistant yeasts. Without routine susceptibility testing of isolates from the high risk compromised population, resistance can be overlooked and treatment failures may be associated with the host's lack of immunological competence rather than the development of Amp-B resistance.

The MFC, the minimal fungicidal concentration, of Amp-B with fungal isolates can be determined with broth techniques. Maybe the MFC data correlate better with the clinical efficacy, especially with patients having leukocyte defects or with granulocytopenic patients. Amp-B is usually fungicidal at achievable levels with very similar inhibitory and fungicidal end points. However, Amp-B tolerance has been reported for isolates of C. parapsilosis[11], some Aspergillus spp., zygomycetes, and other filamentous fungi[1]. Treatment of these infections might require alternative therapeutic approaches.

When should susceptibility testing of fungi to Amp-B be performed? There are a number of incidences when testing may be indicated. Since Amp-B diffuses poorly into body fluids and bone, susceptibility testing may be necessary to insure than an isolate recovered from these sites is highly susceptibile to Amp-B . In some circumstances, the isolation f a fungus from an Amp-B treatment failure or relapse may call for susceptibility testing to insure that the susceptibility of the isolate has not changed during therapy. Isolates of fungal species which may or may not be susceptibile such as Aspergillus or Pseudallescheria boydii, should be tested. Amp-B susceptibility should also be confirmed when an uncommon fungal pathogen is recovered from an opportune infection. This usually occurs in immunocompromised patients, where there are very limited or no susceptibility results available concerning this species. Lastly, the continued emergence of Amp-B resistant yeasts from immunocompromised patients suggests that Amp-B susceptibility should be monitored.

5-Fluorocytosine

Susceptibility testing with 5-FC should be performed more frequently than with Amp-B due to de novo resistance and to the development of resistance during therapy, Broth dilution, disk diffusion, agar dilution[1], and radiometric methods[12] have been developed to assess the in vitro activity of 5-FC with both yeasts and filamentous fungi.

Problems of solubility and stability do not exist with 5-FC testing. However, since 5-FC is an intracellular inhibitor of uracil metabolism and is actively transported into the cell, the presence of cytosine, purines, pyrimidines and nucleosides in the test media can competitively inhibit the uptake of 5-FC and give invalid susceptibility results. In addition, the inoculum size can influence the results when testing yeasts. Generally, there is an increase in resistance when the inoculum size used for the susceptibility test is too high; too small an inoculum may yield false susceptible results.

The spectrum of activity of 5-FC is limited to the de novo resistance of many medically important fungi[1]. The medically important yeasts and certain dematiaceous fungi are generally susceptibile (MIC's $\leq$ 16 µg/ml). De novo resistance can occur with isolates of Candida spp. and Trichosporum beigelii. The agents of the systemic mycoses, Histoplasma capsulatum, Blastomyces dermatidis, Coccidioides immitis, and Paracoccidioides brasiliensis are resistant. Aspergillus spp. and the zygomycetes are usually resistant to 5-FC. the MFC's for many 5-FC susceptible isolates are significantly higher than the MIC, indicating the fungistatic activity of this antifungal agent[1].

Susceptibility testing should be performed on all fungal isolates before initiation of therapy and on all isolates recovered during therapy.

Imidazoles

The newest antifungal agents are the imidazoles, miconazole and ketoconazole. Both alter the cell membrane of fungi by blocking sterol synthesis, although other mechanism(s) may also occur[13]. While both are relatively stable, they are also relatively insoluble in water, requiring polar solvents. Broth dilutions, agar dilution, and disk susceptibility tests have been developed[1], but the validity of in vitro susceptibility data remains unclear. Changes in the basal media used can yield a susceptible or resistant result with a single isolate. Generally, the more enriched the media the more resistant the isolate. Correlation of susceptibility data and clinical efficacy is necessary to determine the validity of the procedures and interpretations. Generally, all yeasts, including Cryptococcus neoformans, agents of systemic mycoses, and some filamentous fungi are considered susceptible with MIC's < 4.0 µg/ml[1]. Concentrations necessary for fungicidal endpoints are usually higher than the MIC's and may limit the usefulness of these agents in treating fungal infections in severely immunocompromised patients. Definition and standardization of in vitro testing and further clinical efficacy studies are necessary before recommendations can be made. At the present time susceptibility testing should probably only be performed on isolates of fungi considered resistant to Amp-B or with fungal isolates from the rare patient who truly cannot tolerate Amp-B . When tests are standardized and the results are correlated with clinical responses, then susceptibility testing may be warranted.

Synergy

Combinations of amphotericin B with other antifungal agents and certain antibacterial antibiotics have been tested in vitro for their antifungal activity. The primary aim of these studies was to find improved therapeutic approaches possibly permitting the decrease in the dosages of Amp-B required, thereby avoiding some toxic reactions. The basis for the use of Amp-B in combination with other agents depends on concentrations of Amp-B, below the MIc, affecting the permeability of the fungal cell membrane, thereby potentiating the uptake of the second agent, increasing the antifungal activity.

Synergistic effects have been demonstrated in vitro with Amp-B in combination with 5-FC, rifampin, and tetracycline. Synergistic or additive effects of Amp-B with 5-FC have been reported[14-22] with medically important yeasts, including Cryptococcus neoformans, and Aspergillus spp. Synergy with Amp-B and rifampin in vitro or in animal models has been noted[22-33] with Candida spp., Aspergillus spp., Coccidioides immitis, Histoplasma capsulatum, and Blastomyces dermatitidis. Synergy with Amp-B and tetracyclines has been noted[23,33] in vitro or with animal models with Coccidioides immitis and Candida albicans. Of all these combinations, only Amp-B with 5-FC used in the treatment of cryptococcal meningitis, has been studied in a controlled clinical trial, showing an improvement in the efficacy of treatment over Amp-B alone[34].

The combined activity of the imidazoles and other antifungal agents has also been investigated. Since miconazole and ketoconazole both affect fungal cell membranes, these antifungals may also potentiate the entry of a second agent. Combinations of miconazole or ketoconazole with 5-FC have been shown[35] to have an additive effect on many isolates of the medically important yeasts and some isolates of Aspergillus fumigatus, as well as synergistic effect on some isolates of the same species.

In vitro susceptibility data on the effects of Amp-B with miconazole or ketoconazole are unclear at the present time. Amp-B with ketoconazole or with miconazole were found[35] to be synergistic or additive with some isolates of Candida spp., Cryptococcus neoformans, and Aspergillus fumigatus, while antagonism was rarely noted with C. albicans and A. fumigatus. However, Candida albicans cells grown in the presence of ketoconazole were shown[36] to be resistant to Amp-B due to the blocking of ergosterol synthesis, implying an unfavorable activity of these 2 antifungal agents. Other studies have reported antagonism[37,38] when using Amp-B combined with miconazole. Lastly, Amp-B with ketoconazole or with miconazole were antagonistic for C. albicans with short incubation times (under 2 hr.), but when the incubation time was increased to 72 hours, an additive effect was noted[39]. the effects ofAmp-B combined with imidazoles remain to be clarified in the face of this conflicting in vitro data, all of which reflect different experimental conditions.

Further in vitro data and studies of the mechanisms of the interactions of antifungl agents are needed to confirm their apparent synergistic effects. Finally, the in vitro data must be correlated with in vivo data to prove the significance of the use of combinations of antifungal agents.

CONCLUSION

The appropriate use of in vitro susceptibility data can aid

in the management of mycoses and individual patients with fungal infections especially in the immunocompromised patients. Standardized procedures, control organisms, and reagents must be defined and confirmed in efficacy studies before in vitro testing will be an accepted procedure. In addition, newer antifungal agents must be developed to provide better approaches to the management of these infections.

ACKNOWLEDGEMENTS

This manuscript would not have been possible without the support of J. Dick, D. Dixon, D. Fay, B. Thumar, and D. Gray.

REFERENCES

1. Shadomy, S. and Espinal-Ingroff, A., in Lennett, E.H., Balows, A., Hausler, W.J. and Truant, J.P. (ed), Manual of Clinical Microbiology, 3rd Ed., p. 647, (1980).
2. Hopfer, R.L. and Groschel, D., Antimicrob. Agents Chemother., 11:277, (1977).
3. Bodenhoff, J., Odontol. Tidskr., 76:276, (1968).
4. Drutz, D.J. and Lehrer, R.I., Amer. J. Med. Sci., 276:77, (1978).
5. Safe, L.M., Safe, S.H., Subden, R.E. and Morris, D.J., Can. J. Microbiol., 23:398, (1977).
6. Pappagianis, D., Collins, M.S., Hector, R. and Remington, J., Antimicrobiol. Agents Chemother., 16:123, (1979).
7. Merz, W.G. and Sandford, G.R., J.Clin. Microbiol., 9:677, (1979).
8. Guinet, R., Chanas, J., Goullier, A., Bonnefoy, G. and Ambroise-Thomas, P., J. Clin. Microbiol., 18:443, (1983).
9. Boyer, J.M., Abstracts of ASM Annual Meeting 1981, p. 320, (1981).
10. Athar, M.A. and Winner, H.I., J. Med. Microbiol., 4:508, (1971).
11. Seidenfeld, S.M., Cooper, B.H., Smith, J.W., Luby, J.P. and Machowiak, P.A., J. Infect. Dis., 147:116, (1983).
12. Hopfer, R.L., Mills, K. and Groschel, D., Antimicrob. Agents Chemother., 15:313, (1979).
13. Taylor, F.R., Rodriguez, R.J. and Parks, L.W., J. Bacteriol., 155:64, (1983).
14. Beggs, W.H., Andrews, F.A. and Sarosi, G.A., Res. Commun. Chem. Pathol. Pharmacol., 16:575, (1977).
15. Dupont, B. and Drouchet, E., Postgrad. Med. J., 55:683, (1979).
16. Fields, B.T., Meredeth, W.R., Galbrath, J.E. and Hardin, H.F., Clin. Res., 22:32a, (1974).

17. Kitahara, M., Seth, V.K., Medoff, G. and Kobayashi, G.S., Antimicrobiol. Agents Chemother., 9:915, (1976).
18. Medoff, G., Comfort, M. and Kobayashi, G.S., Proc. Soc. Exp. Biol. Med., 138:571, (1971).
19. Montgomerie, J.Z., Edwards, J.E. and Guze, L.B., J. Infect. Dis., 132:82, (1971).
20. Medoff, G., Kobayashi, G.S., Kwan, C.N., Schlessinger, D., and Venkov, P., Proc. Natl. Acad. Sci. U.S.A., 69:196, (1972).
21. Polak, A., Bull. Soc. Fr. Mycol. Med., 3:175, (1974).
22. Shadomy, S., Wagner, G., Espinel, Ingrof, A. and Davis, B.A., Antimicrob. Agents Chemother., 8:117, (1974).
23. Ansehn, S., Curr. Ther. Res., 22:92, (1977).
24. Beggs, W.H., Sarosi, G.A. and Andrews, F.A., Amer. Rev. Respir. Dis., 110:671, (1974).
25. Beggs, W.H., Sarosi, G.A. and Walker, M.I., J. Infect. Dis., 133:206, (1976).
26. Dougherty, P.F., Yotter, D.W. and Matthews, T.R., Antimicrob. Agents Chemother., 11:225, (1977).
27. Huppert, M., Pappagianis, D., Sun, S.H., Gleason-Jordan, I., Collins, M.S., and Vukovich, K.R., Antimicrob., 9:406, (1976).
28. Kobayashi, G.S., Cheung, S.C., Schlessinger, D. and Medoff, G., Antimicrob. Agents Chemother., 5:16, (1974).
29. Kobayashi, G.S., Medoff, G., Schlessinger, D., Kwan, C.N. and Musser, W.E., Science, 177:709, (1972).
30. Kwan, C.N., Medoff, G., Kobayashi, G.S., Schlessinger, D. and Raskas, H.J., Antimicrob. Agents Chemother., 2:61, (1972).
31. Medoff, G., Kobayashi, G.S., Kwan, C.N., Schlessinger, D. and Venkov, P., Proc. Natl. Acad. Sci. U.S., 69:196, (1972).
32. Rifkind, D., Crowder, e.D. and Hyland, R.N., Antimicrob. Agents Chemother., 6:783.
33. Lew, M.A., Beckett, K.M. and Levin, M.J., J. Infect. Dis., 136:263, (1977).
34. Bennet, J.E., Dismukes, W.E., Duma, R.J., Medoff, G., Sande, M.A., Gallis, H., Leonard, J., Fields, B.T., Bradshaw, M., Haywood, H., McGee, Z.A., Cate, T.R., Cobb, C.G., Warner, J.F. and Alling, D.W., N. Engl. J. Med., 301:126, (1979).
35. Odds, F.C., Antimicrob. Agents Chemother., 22:763, (1982).
36. Sud, I.J. and Feingold, D.S., Antimicrob. Agents Chemother., 23:185, (1983).
37. Shacter, L.P., Owellen, R.J., Rathbun, H.K., and Buchannan, B., Lancet, 2:318, (1976).
38. Cosgrove, R.F., Beezer, A.E., and Miles, R.J., J.Infect. Dis., 138:681-685, (1976).
39. Brajtburg, J., Kobayashi, D., Medoff, G. and Kobayashi, G.S., J. Infect. Dis., 146:138, (1982).

CRYPTOSPORIDIUM -- BIOLOGY AND DIAGNOSIS

Pearl Ma

Chief of Microbiology
St. Vincent's Hospital & Medical Center of New York
New York, New York

INTRODUCTION

Cryptosporidium species, a minute coccidial protozoan, is a widely publicized causative agent of diarrheal infections in both immunocompromised[1-6] and noncompromised hosts[7-12]. Cryptosporidiosis is characterized by chronic intractable watery diarrhea and abdominal pain. Marked weight loss is often noted in the immunocompromised host especially in patients with acquired immunodeficiency syndrome (AIDS). Cryptosporidial cholecystitis[12-14] and diffuse pneumonia[15-17] have been reported as complications and disseminated cryptosporidiosis has been reported in an infant with congenital double immune deficiency[16]. Other cases of cryptosporidiosis have been described in patients with immune disorders such as hypogammaglobulinemia[18], leukemia[19], and hemophilia[20]. The recent awareness of this infectious agent originated from investigations of the current AIDS epidemic. A high incidence of individuals with AIDS suffer from intractable watery diarrhea which is refractory to all antimicrobial treatments[21-22]. Even parenteral nutrition is unable to replenish the fluid loss resembling that seen in cholera. The search for a causative agent which was originally suspected to be a virus led to the discovery of numerous minute spherical double-walled structures (3-5um) lining the duodenal microvilli as seen by transmission electron microscopy. These structures actually represented the various endogenous stages of a parasite which was identified as a coccidial protozoan called Cryptosporidium species[4,21-22]. A great deal has been learned and published within the last two years[1-17,19-25] indicating that Cryptosporidium is found not only in the immunocompromised host but that it is ubiquitous and has caused travellers' diarrhea[23-24], outbreaks in day care centers[25], nosocomial infections (unpublished data) and community acquired infections in the general populations [9-11,28,57]. The mode of transmission is most likely oral-fecal with a high incidence of person to person spread[3,22,6], water/food borne transmission[23], and animal contact in special settings[6]. Respiratory cryptosporidiosis due to inhalation of oocysts may be another mode of transmission[15,17]. The prevalance of cryptosporidiosis varies from approximately 4%-10% in normal individuals[28,8-11] to 28% in homosexuals and bisexuals, with 18% in AIDS and 10% in non-AIDS non-compromised individuals[12]. The purpose of this chapter is to present briefly the biology (general characteristics, life cycle) and the diagnosis (clinical and microbiological) of Cryptosporidium species for those who are not familiar with this parasite.

BIOLOGY

General Characteristics of Cryptosporidium

Cryptosporidium species was discovered and classified by Professor E.E. Tyzzer, head of the Department of Comparative Parasitology, Harvard School of Medicine in 1907 when he examined the gastric tumor of a house-mouse and was surprised to find numerous minute parasites (3-5um) unknown to anyone at that time[26]. By examining the intestinal sections with touch preparations stained with various stains he identified the parasite as a protozoan belonging to the Coccidia. The taxonomy of Cryptosporidium sp. as related to other members of the Coccidia is shown in Figure 1[27].

Cryptosporidium As a Single Species

From 1907 to 1981, Cryptosporidium has been found to be the causative agent of diarrhea in mammals and invertebrates, respiratory and intestinal infections in birds, and disseminated disease in immunocompromised arabian foals and juvenile monkeys[1,28]. From 1976-1981, only 6 cases were reported in humans[1,28]. Due to the lack of information of the complete life cycle, it was believed that there existed various species of Cryptosporidium depending on the host it affected[27]. Levine recommended that of the 19 species named previously, only four could be considered valid (C. muris, Tyzzer, 1907, in mammals; C. meleagridis, Slavin, 1955, in birds; C. crotali, Triffit, 1925 in reptiles; and C. nasorum, Hoover, Hoerr, Carlton, Hinsman & Ferguson, 1981 in fish)[29].

In 1980, Tzipori et al conducted cross infections of Cryptosporidium among different mammals such as lamb, calf[30], and pig[31], and established the existence of a single species[32]. This was confirmed by other investigators[6,33].

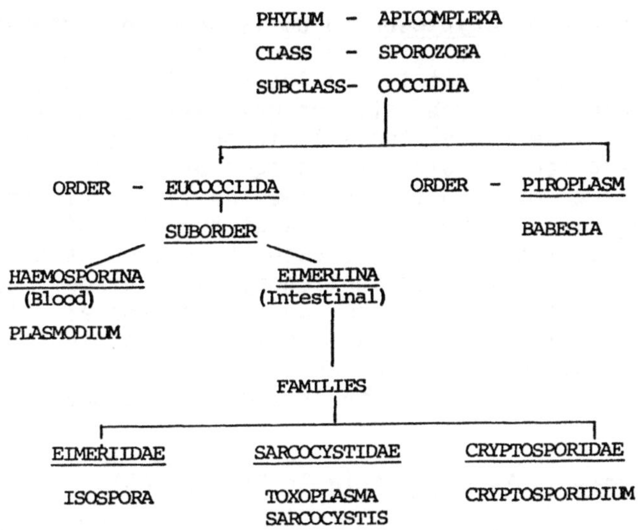

Fig. 1. Classification of *Cryptosporidium* as related to other members of the Coccidia

Whether this single species is also found in birds and reptiles will await further investigation.

LIFE CYCLE

The life cycle is very similar to other members of the coccidial protozoans, as there is an alternation of asexual and sexual reproduction. In *Plasmodium* (malarial parasite), the asexual life cycle takes place within the human erythrocytes while the sexual life cycle occurs in another host, the female Anopheles mosquito. *Cryptosporidium* , unlike *Plasmodium*, has both life cycles completed in the intestinal enterocytes in one host (monoxenous), as occurs in another coccidium, *Isospora* species. However, *Cryptosporidium* differs from *Isospora* in being extracytoplasmic while *Isospora* is intracytoplasmic. Therefore, *Cryptosporidium* is usually regarded as a non-invasive organism, while *Isopora* is invasive. At least this is the state of the art as we now know it[34,58].

The life cycle of Cryptosporidium is depicted schematically in Figure 2. The complete life cycle was not known until 1979 when Iseki[34] demonstrated it in the intestinal mucosa as well as in the fecal material of the cat. As one reviews the literature of the coccidial life cycle, there is inconsistency in the use of the terms to describe the different stages of the coccidial protozoans. The terms used to describe the life cycle of Cryptosporidium will be those in vogue at the time of this writing[35,37]. For instance, terms such as merogony and merozoites are used instead of schizogony and schizont; gamonts refer to the early stages of micro- and macro-gametes. The microgamont gives rise to microgametocyte which divides to give rise to 14 microgametes while in the case of the macrogamont, it becomes the macrogamete, hence the term macrogametocyte is not applicable[37].

Asexual Life Cycle -- Merogony (Fig 2: Stages 1-5)

The cryptosporidial oocyst is the infective stage (7S). Upon ingestion by the host, it undergoes excystation in the presence of trypsin and bile in the stomach, liberating the four banana-shaped sporozoites, each of which attaches itself to the surface membrane of the host enterocyte by the blunt nucleated end without entering the cytoplasm (Stage 1). Soon it rounds up to become a trophozoite (T) enclosed within a parasitophorous vacuole consisting of four unit membranes. (Stage 2). The outer two membranes are presumed to be of host origin while the inner ones originated from the parasite. A thick band of attachment (AB) is visible between the parasite and the host[34,36],. This has been an area of controversy among various investigators since some demonstrated that the organism is extracellular[26,28], while others presented evidence that it is intracellular[36] but extracytoplasmic[34]. The trophozoite measuring 3.8 x 3.7 um[37] undergoes mitotic divisions to form two, four and then eight banana-shaped merozoites. This is called the Type I meront (ME-I) which is larger than the trophozoite, measuring 5.2 x 5.1 um[37] (Stages 3 & 4). At maturity, the merozoites are liberated. They attach themselves to the surrounding uninfected microvilli (MV) and the asexual cycle repeats itself (Stage 5). This may explain the situation of how an immunosuppressed patient with congenital hypogammaglobulinemia could develop a chronic infection following an initially acquired exogenous infection[18].

The Sexual Life Cycle -- Gametogony (Fig 2: Stages 1S-7S)

At some point the merozoite (Stage 1S), instead of repeating the asexual cycle, rounds up to become the trophozoite (Stage 2S). It undergoes divisions to form four merozoites (Stage 3S) instead of eight as the Type I meront in the asexual cycle shown above. This gives rise to the Type II meront (ME-II) measuring

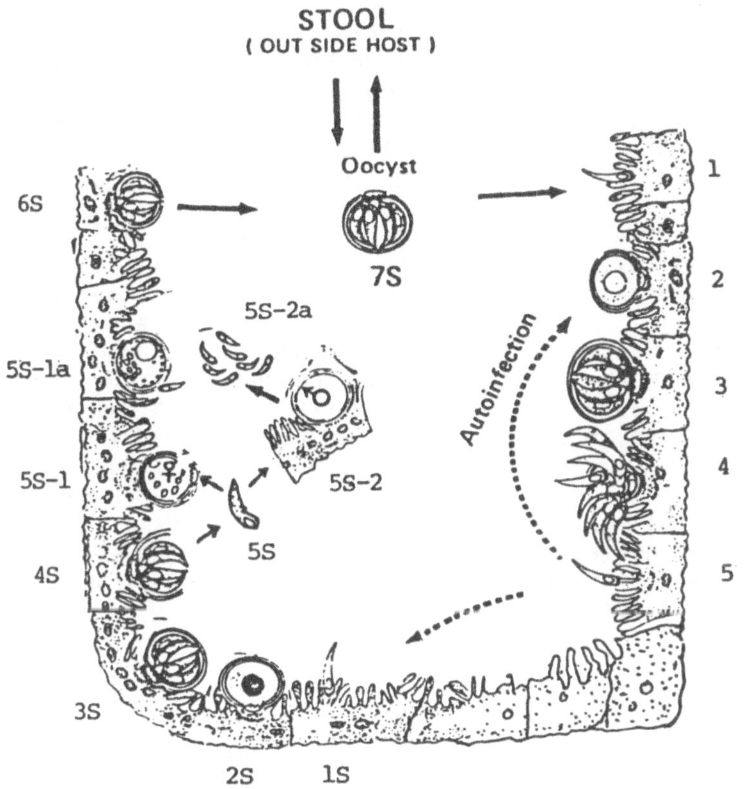

SEXUAL	ASEXUAL
1S- Sporozoite	1- Sporozoite
2S- Trophozoite	2- Trophozoite
3S- Type II meront	3- Type I meront
4S- Type II merozoite	4- Type I merozoite
5S- Gamont	5- Type I merozoite attached to microvilli
5S- 1-Macrogamont	
5S- 2-Microgametocyte → Microgamont	
5S-1a-Microgamete in contact with macrogamete	
5S-2a-Microgamete	
6S- Zygote becoming an oocyst with 4 banana-shaped sporozoites	
7S- Matured oocyst	

Fig. 2. Schematic Life Cycle of Cryptosporidium Sp.

4.5 x 4.3 um, slightly smaller than the Type I meront (Stage 4S). The Type II merozoite, when liberated, undergoes differentiation to become the female gamont (Stage 5S-1) and the male gamont (Stage 5S-2). The macrogamont matures to become the macrogamete (5.3 x 5.2 um), and is characterized by the presence of numerous polysaccharide granules (PG) (Stage 5S-1a). The male gamont matures to become the microgametocyte (4.5 x 4.5 um) which gives rise to 14 minute microgametes (Stage 5S-2a). The microgametes are not flagellated but they glide towards the macrogamete where fertilization takes place (Stage 5S-1a). A zygote is formed and is surrounded by a double wall to produce the oocyst (5.2 x 5.4 um) (Stage 6S). At maturity, the oocyst gives rise to four naked banana-shaped sporozoites without a sporocyst. The sporulated oocyst is then extruded into the lumen and is found in the fecal material (Stage 7S). It has been postulated that two types of oocysts exist. The thin-walled one excysts in the host and repeats the sexual life cycle, while the thick walled one is extruded into the intestinal lumen and finds itself in the fecal material[37].

Some of the endogenous stages described above are shown in the Transmission electron micrographs, the scanning electron micrographs and light microscopy and the fluorescent and light microscopy of oocysts.

CLINICAL DIAGNOSIS

The natural history of cryptosporidiosis is not well known. As we know from some of our cases, the incubation period may vary from one to twelve days. The mode of transmission is most likely oral-fecal with a high incidence of person to person spread.[10,11] Other modes suggest sexual transmission in the homosexual and bisexual population[3,21,22] and water/food borne transmission in traveller's diarrhea[8,23-24]. Transmission from animals is more likely to occur in a setting such as in rural areas or animal centers[6]. The symptoms of enteritis vary mostly in severity and time span among the immunocompetent versus the immunocompromised hosts with cryptosporidiosis. In the immunocompetent individual who has no underlying disease, the symptoms are marked by watery diarrhea varying from 3-10 times of bowel movements representing 1-3 liters/day. The accompanying symptoms include abdominal pain, nausea, vomiting, flatulence, fever, headache, dehydration in descending order of frequency [1-2,6-12]. The stool is non-bloody, with/without mucus and without fecal leukocytes unless invasive enteric pathogen(s) are present. Incubation period, if known, varies from 1-12 days, median 6-7 days. Duration of diarrhea varies from 1-30 days, median 12-14 days. In general, the symptoms are more severe in children than in adults[28,24,10].

Usually no hospitalization is necessary except when other enteric pathogens are present such as Salmonella, Shigella, Campylobacter, E. histolytica or Giardia[7,24,9,25].

In the immunocompromised host, as in the case of AIDS or in individuals with other immune disorders[18-20], the symptoms are more chronic, lasting 3 years--as seen in a child with hypogammaglobulinemia[18]. Moreover, many months of intractable watery diarrhea[1-6,13-17,21-22] can occur, with marked weight loss up to 70 lbs in AIDS patients. Daily bowel movements vary from 5-25 times/day with fluid loss from 1-10 liters/day. Numerous anti-parasitic drugs have failed to alleviate the symptoms significantly[1,28]. Spiramycin has given various clinical and parasitological responses[38]. In our group of AIDS patients treated with spiramycin, clinical responses were minimal and upon cessation of treatment the patient's diarrheal condition continued to deteriorate. The parasitological response was short-lived with a slight drop in the number of oocysts for the first few days during treatment followed by an increase of oocysts in the stool. This response may be related to the immune deficiency state of the patient (unpublished data).

Complications
(Cholecytitis, diffuse pneumonia and disseminated cryptosporidiosis)

Severe intestinal cryptosporidiosis may lead to fatal complications in immunocompromised hosts. One complication of intestinal cryptosporidiosis involved the gall-bladder causing cholecystitis[12-14] with/without acalculous gangrene[13]. The patient suffered from upper quadrant pain and had an elevated alkaline phosphatase. Diffuse pneumonia with/without cough and copious white sputum was an additional complication of cryptosporidiosis in humans[15-17]. The most severe complication of cryptosporidiosis was a case of disseminated disease reported in one infant with combined immune deficiencies[16].

LABORATORY DIAGNOSIS

Stool Examination for Diarrheal Diseases

When a patient suffering from diarrhea seeks medical help, the clinicians require the clinical microbiology laboratory to aid in establishing the diagnosis. Whether it is bacterial, viral or parasitic, a fresh stool specimen is preferred. The same specimen can be processed for bacterial culture (Salmonella, Shigella, Campylobacter, Yersinia, Aeromonas, Mycobacteria, etc.), for viral culture or detection of viral antigen (Adenovirus, Rotavirus, etc) and ova and parasites (Cryptosporidium, Entamoeba histolytica,

Giardia lamblia, helminths, etc.). Concomitant infections with bacteria, parasites and viruses are not infrequent, especially in AIDS patients. Since these patients are frequently treated with multiple antibiotics for their opportunistic infections, *Clostridium difficile* toxin should also be included in the diagnostic testing. Therefore it is good practice to cover the above tests if the situation allows. If the clinical laboratory is set up so that the parasitiology laboratory is separate from the other parts of the Microbiology laboratory, then it will require separate specimens. From 1976-1981, diagnosis of cryptosporidiosis was based primarily on intestinal or rectal biopsies using electron microscopy[39]. The minute 3-5μm spherical structures attach to the intestinal enterocytes causing atrophic microvilli, stunting and fusion with epithelial cross-bridges between adjacent villi.

In 1981, Tzipori diagnosed the first human cryptosporidiosis by stool examination, using Giemsa stained fecal smears to reveal the cryptosporidial oocysts[40]. Now it has become the standard diagnostic method since it allows one to screen a large volume of specimens without invasive procedures. Henricksen further improved the methodology of stool examination by introducing the Ziehl-Neelsen acid fast fecal smear showing that the cryptosporidial oocysts are acid fast and are easy to detect or to differentiate from yeasts which resemble the oocysts in size and morphology[41,4]. By adopting a more rapid method of the Modified Cold Kinyoun (MCK) Procedure, the staining time can be drastically reduced from 30 mins to 1 min simply by supplementing the carbol fuchsin with 1% tergitol[4,25]. Tergitol is a surface acting agent which reduces the surface tension of the oocyst wall and allows easy penetration of the carbol fuchsin in a short time. However, in formalin fixed fecal smear, the staining time has to be extended to 5-10 min due to the fixed oocyst wall. In this case both carbol fuchsin with/without tergitol can be used although the stain without tergitol gives better result. One also needs a strong decolorizer (10% H_2SO_4) since various fecal materials will be stained by the carbol fuchsin and will present difficulties in identifying the acid-fast oocyst. The life cycle of *Cryptosporidium* requires approximately 4-5 days, thus the number of oocysts present in the stool specimen depends on the degree of oocyst shedding. In highly suspected cases, at least 3 specimens should be examined within a 5 day period before it is regarded as negative. In some specimens, especially the semi-solid or formed stools, the number of oocysts may not be high, hence concentration procedures are needed to have an accurate result of the stool examination. Anderson[42] used the sucrose flotation procedure to facilitate the concentration of oocysts, especially in specimens with low numbers of organisms, while Iseki[34] used zinc sulphate flotation. Both procedures should work well to concentrate the oocysts which are extremely light requiring a medium such as sucrose or zinc sulphate solution with a high specific gravity to allow the oocyst to float. On the other hand, if the stool is semi-solid the presence of fecal material may be able to concentrate the oocysts during centrifugation, this is not satisfactory in the watery stool without much fecal material. In AIDS patients, the common consistency of the stool is pure liquid devoid of fecal material[4], hence flotation will be more highly desirable to centrifugation procedure. It has been found that the ether/ethyl-acetate used in the standard formalin-ether/ethyl acetate concentration procedure[43] will cause some of the oocysts to lose the acid fastness and may lead to false negative results (unpublished data).

To incorporate new procedures in a busy clinical parasitology laboratory, the goal is to utilize existing laboratory procedures and to adopt a rapid test to reduce turn-around time as well as have a permanent record of the specimen examination for future reference especially for confirmation of treatment cases. Pseudo-epidemics of amebiasis are well-know due to faulty techniques of parasitic examination; similar events should be avoided in the laboratory diagnosis of cryptosporidiosis[44]. Frequently we receive specimens from various sources for confirmation of cryptosporidiosis and it is not surprising to see a high incidence of false positive laboratory diagnoses of cryptosporidiosis due to inadequate decolorization, misreading of yeasts, or artifacts, mistaken for cryptosporidial oocysts. Additionally, false negative results occur because the specimens were not concentrated by sugar flotation or centrifugation.

Electron microscopy and histological sectioning of biopsied material for cryptosporidiosis will not be dealt with here since numberous publications are available[36,34,45-47].

<u>Stool Examinations for Intestinal Cryptosporidiosis</u>

Various methodologies have been available in the literature for the stool examination for cryptosporidia[4,48-53]. Space will not allow for review all of them here. However, the methods familiar to us which have proven to be effective will be presented. Conventional methods such as the saline and iodine preparations for the detection of ova and parasites are supplemented with specific procedures such as the modified cold kinyoun (MCK), sucrose direct preparation and sucrose flotation procedures in our routine three-step stool examination for Cryptosporidiosis[4,53]. The reagents needed are listed in the Appendix.

Since December 1981, more than 100 cases of intestinal, four biliary, and five respiratory, cryptosporidiosis have been diagnosed in our laboratory[1-4,12,15,17,21,23,24,53].

Iodine Wet Preparation -- One drop of D'Antoine iodine used to examine amoebic cysts can be added to one drop of fecal material (fresh/preserved specimen). Cryptosporidial oocysts remain unstained while amoeba and yeasts will stain brown by the iodine[4].

Sucrose Wet Preparation -- One drop of sucrose used in the sucrose flotation procedure can be added to a drop of fecal material on a slide covered with a cover-slip. By examining the preparation under an American-Optic microscope (AO) or the Nikon Laboflot microscope, under the low/high power objectives, the oocysts appear with a pink hue while yeasts will not[4,1]. This is not specific for cryptosporidia since *Isospora*, *Eimeria* and *Giardia* cysts also appear pink. However, one can easily differentiate them by their size and morphology[53]. Sucrose can cause indentation leading to rupture of the oocysts upon standing, hence the preparation is best examined within 15 min.

Modified Cold Kinyoun (MCK) Preparation. There are two methods to perform the acid fast staining procedures, one is the rapid 1 min stained procedure for unpreserved stools and the other is the 5-10 min staining for preserved specimens.

Rapid 1 min MCK for unpreserved stool[4,53].

a. Prepare a thin fecal smear, and air dry
b. Fix in absolute methanol for a few seconds
c. Flood slide with carbol fuchsin supplemented with 1% tergitol.
d. Let stand for 1 min.
e. Rinse thoroughly in tap water until no pink color elutes.
f. Drain excess water.
g. Dip in 10% H_2SO_4 for a few seconds.
h. Rinse immediately in tap water to prevent overdecolorization.
i. Drain excess water.
j. Dip in conc light green or methylene blue for a few seconds.
k. Rinse well in tap water.
l. Blot dry and read under low/high/oil objectives for acid fast (red) oocysts.
   Low power -- pinpoint red structures
   High power -- 4-5um acid fast spherical structures
   Oil immersion lens -- 4-5 um spherical structures with or without a minute round residual body. Banana-shaped sporozoites may be visible in some preparations. The cyst wall is usually not stained and appears as a halo around the oocyst. In any preparation, one can see some

oocysts stained deep red, some with black granules, some stained pink and some light pink and some unstained. This may be due to the length of staining time, or to the condition of the oocyst in the population, or even to the maturity of the oocyst present in the fecal specimen. Young oocysts attached to the micro-villi are less acid fast than those extruded into the intestinal lumen when they reach maturity. In severe infections, less mature stages may be shed into the intestinal lumen and appear non-acid fast. At least one can see the unstained oocyst on the smear, while in the Truant's auramine-rhodamine smear, it will be completely invisible. Further work is underway to determine the basis for the staining characteristics.

5-10 Min MCK for Preserved Specimens. Follow above procedure except carbol fuchsin without tergitol in Step c will give better results, and the staining time in Step d is extended to 5-10 min.

Fluorescent Staining. There are two methods available. One is the Fluorochrome Truant auramine-rhodamine stain used to stain *Mycobacteria*[43]. A modification of this is the use of phenol auramine-carbol fuchsin double stain which gives good results[49]. The other is the indirect fluorescent antibody test by using the intestinal tissue section containing the organisms[54-55] or fecal oocysts as the source of antigen[56] for determining the anti-cryptosporidial antibody level.

Truant's Stain for *Cryptosporidium*

a. Prepare fecal smear as above.
b. Flood slide with auramine-rhodamine stain for 15 min.
c. Rinse in tap water.
d. Decolorize with 0.5% HCl in 70% ethyl alcohol for 2-3 min.
e. Rinse in tap water.
f. Flood slide with counterstain 0.5% aqueous potassium permanganate for 2-3 min to render background nonfluorescent
g. Rinse, dry, and examine with an ultra-violet scope equipped with BG 12 excitation filter and a barrier filter OG1, or the G filter in the Nikon Laboflot equipped with fluorescence.

Oocyst -- bright yellow fluorescence with a black background. Some may appear light green
Yeast -- Light green or invisible

As shown above with MCK, not all oocysts in any preparation will be detected. When they fail to fluoresce and appear green, they may be confused with yeasts, or if they are invisible, they will be missed completely.

Modified Truant's Stain with MCK for Cryptosporidium. The use of fluorescent scope which is adapted so that the same field can be changed to bright light will allow one to confirm whether the organism is an oocyst by using a smear stained with Truant's stain as above, followed by 1 min MCK. We saw oocysts which were stained acid fast with MCK but failed to fluoresce with Truant's stain.

In other words, no one method of staining is 100% effective. One has to choose the one which is most ideal for the individual laboratory setting/expertise. On the other hand, the different degrees of staining might very well be due to the biological characteristics of the different stages of the organism.

Indirect fluorescent antibody test (IFAT). Antigen from tissue infected with cryptospordia[55,56]/antigen from fecal oocysts[57] have been used to measure elevated anti-cryptosporidial titer[23,24].

Concentration Procedures for Cryptosporidium

Sucrose flotation procedure.

a. Stool is filtered through 2 pieces of square gauze.
b. Place 2 ml of fecal suspension in a 15ml conical centrifuge tube.
c. Add sucrose solution until it is 2/3 full.
d. With a few wooden applicators, break up the large particles to free the oocysts.
e. Fill the tube with sucrose, leaving 2-3 cm from the top.
f. Cap the tube well.
g. Centrifuge at 1,000 rpm for 10 min.
h. Remove the cap. A loopful of surface material can be placed on a slide with a coverslip for examination or one can top the tube with more sucrose forming a convex surface so that a coverslip placed on top of it will allow the oocysts to float to the coverslip. After 10-15 min standing at room temperature, the coverslip can be placed on a slide for examination. The oocysts appear 4-5um with a pink hue with/without a minute residual body. Some oocysts may appear indented dueto the sucrose pushing on the oocyst wall, leading to rupture upon standing. Hence, the preparation should be read within 30 min. Yeast will not appear with a pink hue.

Zinc sulphate flotation method[34]

Modified Formalin-ether concentration[43]. Proceed to the step where ether is to be added, make a smear with the sediment and observe it with the direct sucrose preparation or stain with MCK or Truant's stain. Ether will cause the oocysts to lose acid fastness. Therefore, it should not be added for using acid fast staining for cryptosporidia.

Intestinal Biopsy

The mature oocysts are usually located on the surface of the biopsy and therefore it should not be rinsed before touch preparation is made. Touch preparation is prepared by using the cut surface of the tissue and by touching the surface of a clean slide at several different sites. Fix with absolute methanol and proceed to stain with MCK for 1 min or 10 min as above.

Biliary & Respiratory Cryptosporidiosis

An immunocompromised host who suffers from intestinal cryptosporidiosis for more than one month may develop complications with cryptosporidiosis in the respiratory or biliary tract. Specimens such as bronchial alveolar lavage or sputum can be used to prepare a direct or concentrated smear as one processes the specimen for tubercle bacilli and proceed with the staining with the 1 min/10 min MCK; sucrose preparation or Truant's stain.

For an open lung biopsy, proceed as with intestinal biopsy above. It is important to do a duplicate smear stained for *Pneumocystis carinii* in the AIDS population. In our laboratory, the 1 min Hemacolor stain procedure give immediate results[15,53].

CONCLUSION

In conclusion, *Cryptosporidium* species, a minute coccidial protozoan has been presented as a new infectious agent causing diarrhea not only in the immunocompromised host but also causing self-limited diarrhea in immuno-competent individuals--as in traveller's diarrhea, outbreaks in day care centers, and in the homosexual and bisexual populations. The biology and the diagnoses have been presented. The laboratory procedures are those practiced in our clinical laboratory and can be easily instituted for the accurate diagnosis of both intestinal and respiratory cryptosporidiosis. Other staining procedures are worth trying, but the above regimens have been working effectively in our clinical laboratory with a positive yield of 110 cases of intestinal cryptosporidiosis, 4 cases of cholecystitis and 5 cases of respiratory cryptosporidiosis from 1981-1985.

ACKNOWLEDGEMENT

Research support grant #I120674-02, Prevalence and Pathogenesis of Cryptosporidium , National Institutes of Health, National Institute of Allergy and Infectious Diseases, and the research and clinical microbiology staffs at St. Vincent's Hospital & Medical Center of New York for their excellent technical assistance.

REFERENCES

1. Navin, T.R., Juranek, D.D., Cryptosporidiosis: Clinical, epidemiologic and parasitologic review, Rev. Infect. Dis. 6:313-327 (1984).
2. Marsden, P.D., Ma, P., Human Intestinal Coccidiosis in The Acquired Immune Deficiency Syndrome and Infections in Homosexual Men. (P. Ma and D. Armstrong Eds), Chapter 8, pp 86-94, Yorke Medical Books, New York (1984).
3. Ma, P., (Editorial), Cryptosporidium and the Enteropathy of Immune Deficiency, J. Ped Gastroenterol. & Nutrition. 3:488 (1984).
4. Ma, P., Soave, R., Thee-step stool examination for Cryptosporidiosis in 10 homosexual men with protracted watery diarrhea, J. Infect. Dis. 147:824-828, (1983).
5. Pitlik, S.D., Fainstein, V., Garza, et al., Human Cryptosporidiosis: spectrum of disease. Report of six cases and review of the literature, Arch. Intern. Med. 143: 269-2275 (1983).
6. Current, W.L., Reese, N.C., Ernst, H.V., et al., Human Cryptosporidiosis in immunocompetent and immunodeficient persons, N. Eng. J. Med. 308:1252-1257 (1983).
7. Tzipori, S., Smith, M., Birch, C. et al., Cryptosporidiosis in hospital patients with gastroenteritis, Am. J. Trop. Med. Hyg. 32:931-934 (1983).
8. Jokipii, L. Pohjola, S., Jokipii, A.M., Cryptosporidium: a frequent finding in patients with gastrointestinal symptoms. Lancet II 358-361 (1983).
9. Hunt, D.A., Shannon, R., Palmer, S.R., et al., Cryptosporidiosis in an urban community, Brit. Med. J. 289:814-816 (1984).
10. Mata, L., Bolanos, H., Pizarro, D., et al., Cryptosporidiosis in children from some highland Costa Rican rural and urban areas, Am.J. Trop. Med. Hyg. 33:24-29 (1984).
11. Bogaerts, J., Lepage, P., Rouvroy, D., et al., Cryptosporidium spp., a frequent cause of diarrhea in Central Africa, J.Clin. Microbiol. 20:874-876 (1984).

12. Ma, P., Guigli, P., Kaufman, D., et al., Intestinal and respiratory Cryptosporidiosis in AIDS individuals in New York areas, Abstract 61, p. 100, 24th Interscience Conf. on Antimicrob. Agents & Chemother., Washington D.C. Oct 8 (1984).
13. Blumberg, R.S., Kelsey, P., Perrone, T., et al., Cytomegalovirus--and Cryptosporidium -associated acalculous gangrenous cholecystitis, A.J. Med. 76:1118-1123 (1984).
14. Guarda, L.A., Stein, S.A., Cleary, K.A., et al., Human Cryptosporidiosis in the Acquired Immune Deficiency Syndrome, Arch. Pathol. Lab. Med. 107:562-566 (1983).
15. Ma, P., Villanueva, T.G., Kaufman, D., Gillooley, J.F., Respiratory Cryptosporidiosis in the Acquired Immune Deficiency Syndrome, JAMA 252:1298-1301 (1984).
16. Kocoshis, S.A., Cibull, M.L., Davis, T.E., et al., Intestina l and pulmonary cryptosporidiosis in an infant with severe combined immune deficiency, J. Pediat. Gastroenterol. Nutr. 3:149-157 (1984).
17. Forgacs, P., Tarshis, A., Ma, P. et al., Intestinal and bronchial Cryptosporidiosis in an immunodeficient homosexual man, Ann. Intern. Med. 99:793-794 (1983).
18. Lasser, K.H., Lewin, K.J., Ryning, F.W., Cryptosporidial enteritis in a patient with congenital hypogammaglobl inemia, Human Pathol. 10:234-240 (1979).
19. Miller, R.A., Holmberg, R.E., Clausen, C.R., Life-threatening diarrhea caused by Cryptosporidium in a child undergoing therapy for acute lymphocytic leukemia, J. Ped. 103:256-259 (1983).
20. Koch, K.L., Shankey, T.V., Weinstein, G. et al., Cryptosporidiosis in a patient with hemophilia, common variable hypogammaglobulinemia, and the Acquired Immunodeficiency Syndrome, Annals Intern. Med. 99:337-340 (1983).
21. Ma, P., Soave, R., Cryptosporidiosis, a new enteric coccidiosis emerged as an opportunistic infection in five male homosexuals. (Abstract # 848). In Program and abstracts of the 22nd Interscience Conference on Antimicrobial Agents and Chemotherapy. American Society for Microbiology, Washington, D.C. (1982).
22. Centers for Disease Control, Cryptosporidiosis: assessment of chemotherapy of males with acquired immune deficiency symdrome, MMWR 31:589-592 (1982).
23. Ma, P., Kaufman, D., Helmick, C.G., D'Souza, A.J., Navin, T.R., Cryptosporidiosis in tourists returning from the Carribbean, N. Eng. J. Med. 312:647-648 (1985).
24. Soave, R., Ma, P., Cryptosporidiosis -- traveler's diarrhea in two families, Arch. Intern. Med. 145:70-72 (1985).

25. Centers for Disease Control, Cryptosporidiosis among children attending day-care centers -- Georgia, Pennsylvania, Michigan, California, New Mexico, MMWR 33:599-601 (1984).
26. Tyzzer, E.E., A sporozoon found in the peptic gland of the common mouse, Proc. Soc. Exp. Biol. Med. 5:12 (1907-1908).
27. Levine, N.D., Taxonomy and life cycles of Coccidia in The Biology of Coccidia (Long, P.L., ed.), University Park Press, Baltimore, Chapter 1, pp 33 (1982).
28. Tzipori, S., Cryptosporidiosis in animals and humans, Microbiol. Rev. 47:84-96 (1983).
29. Levine, N.D., Taxonomy and review of the Coccidian genus Cryptosporidium (Protozoa, Apicomplexa), J. Protozool. 31:94-98 (1984).
30. Tzipori, S., Angus, K.W., Gray, E.W., et al., Diarrhea in lambs experimentally infected with Cryptosporidium isolated from calves, Am. J. Vet. Res. 42:1400-1404 (1981).
31. Tzipori, S., McCartney, E., Lawson, G. H., et al., Experimental infection of piglets with Cryptosporidium , Res. in Vet. Sci. 31:358-368 (1981).
32. Tzipori, S., Angus, K.W., Campbell, I., et al., Cryptosporidium : evidence for a single species genus, Infect. Immun. 30:884-886 (1980).
33. Moon, H.W., Bemrick, W.J., Fecal transmission of calf cryptosporidia between calves and pigs, Vet. Pathol. 18:248-255 (1981).
34. Iseki, M., Cryptosporidium felis sp n (Protozoa Eimeriorina) from the domestic cat, Japan J. Parasitol. 28: 285-307 (1979).
35. Chobotar, B., Scholtyseck, E., Ultrastructure in The Biology of the coccidia, (Long, P.L., ed.), University Park Press, Baltimore, Chapter 4, pp. 101-166 (1982).
36. Vetterling, J.M., Takeuchi, A., Madden, P.A., Ultrastructure of Cryptosporidium wrairi from the guinea pig, J. Protozool. 18:248-260 (1971).
37. Current, W.L., Long, P.L., Development of human and calf Cryptosporidium in chicken embryos, J. Infect. Dis 148:1108-1113 (1983).
38. Centers for Diseases Control, Update: treatment of Cryptosporidiosis in patients with acquired immunodeficiency symdrome (AIDS), MMWR 33:117-119 (1984).
39. Weinstein, L., Edelstein, S.M., Madara, J.L., et al., Intestinal Cryptosporidiosis complicated by disseminated Cytomegalovirus infection, Gastroenter. 81:584-591 (1981).
40. Tzipori, S., Angus, K.W., Gray, E.W., Campbell, I., (Letter to the editor), Vomiting and diarrhea associated with Cryptosporidial infection, N. Eng. J. Med. 303:818 (1980).
41. Henriksen, S.A., Pohlenz, J. F., (Brief communication), Staining of Cryptosporidia by a modified Ziehl-Neelsen technique, Acta. vet. scand. 22:594-596 (1981).

42. Anderson, B.C., Patterns of shedding of cryptosporidial oocysts in Idaho calves, J. Am. Vet. Med. Assoc. 178:982-984 (1981).
43. Paik, G., Suggs, M.T., Reagents, stains and miscellaneous test procedures, in Manual of Clinical Microbiology, 2nd ed., (Lennette, Spauding, Truant, eds.), American Society for Microbiology, Washington D.C., Chapter 96, p 930-950 (1974).
44. Centers for Disease Control, Pseudo-outbreak of intestinal amebiasis, MMWR 34:125-126 (1985).
45. Pearson, G.R., Logan, E.F., Scanning and transmission electron microscopic observations on the host-parasite relationship in intestinal Cryptosporidiosis of neonatal calves, Res. in Vet. 34:149-154 (1983).
46. Bird, R.G., Smith, M.D., Cryptosporidiosis in man: parasite life cycle and fine structural pathology, J. Pathol. 132:217-233 (1980).
47. Pohlenz, J., Bemrick, J., Moon, H.W., et al., Bovine Cryptosporidiosis : a transmission and scanning electron microscopic study of some stages in the life cycle and of the host-parasite relationship, Acta. Pathol. 15:417-427 (1978).
48. Garcia, L.S., Bruckner, D.A., Brewer, T.C., et al., Techniques for the recovery and identification of Cryptosporidium oocysts from stool specimens, J. Clin. Microbiol. 18:185-190 (1983).
49. Casemore, D.P., Armstrong, M., Jackson, B., Screening for Cryptosporidium in stools, The Lancet I:734-735 (1984).
50. Baxby, D., Blundell, N., Sensitive, rapid, simple methods for detecting Cryptosporidium in feces, The Lancet II:1149 (1983).
51. Bronsdon, M.A., Rapid dimethyl sulfoxide-modified acid-fast stain of Cryptosporidium oocysts in stool specimens, J. Clin. Microbiol. 19:952-953 (1984).
52. Heine, J., Eine einfache Nachweismethod for Kryptosporidian im Kot zentra (b) Veterinarmed [B] 29:324 (1982).
53. Ma, P., Laboratory diagnosis of coccidiosis in Microbioogy 1984, (L. Leive & D. Schessinger, eds.), American Society for Microbiology, Washington, D.C., p 224-230 (1984).
54. Tzipori, S., Campbell, I., Prevalence of Cryptosporidium antibodies in 10 animal species, J. Clin. Microbiol. 14: 455-456 (1981).
55. Campbell, P.N., Current, W.L., Demonstration of serum antibodies to Cryptosporidium sp. in normal and immunodeficient humans with confirmed infections, J. Clin. Microbiol. 18:165-169 (1983).

56. Tsaihong, J., Ma, P., Identification of fecal cryptosporidial oocysts by comparing sucrose wet preparation modified cold Kinyoun stain and indirect fluorescent tet. (Abstract C 85) in Proceeding and Abstract of the 84th Annual Meeting of the American Society for Microbiology, Washington, D.C. (1984).

57. Ma, P., Cryptosporidiosis in Immune Enteropathy. (A Review) in current Clinical Topics in Infectious Disease. Volume JS Remington & MN Swartz (eds). McGraw-Hill Book Co. In Press. 1986.

58. Ma, P., Kaufman, D., Montana, J., Isospora belli diarrheal Infection in Homosexual Men. AIDS Research 1, #5, 327-33B, 1984.

PNEUMOCYSTIS CARINII PNEUMONIA

David L. Kaufman

Department of Medicine
St. Vincent's Hospital & Medical Center of New York
New York, New York

INTRODUCTION

Prior to 1981, Pneumocystis carinii pneumonia (PCP) was a rather rare disease seen primarily by physicians working with oncology or transplant patients. Then early in June 1981, the Centers for Disease Control (CDC) issued the first report of PCP in five homosexual men in Los Angeles[1]. That brief report, in retrospect, marked the beginning of a new and devastating epidemic -- the Acquired Immune Deficiency Syndrome (AIDS). It was followed, almost weekly, by new reports, papers and conferences that documented the magnitude and lethality of this new syndrome. As of 3/19/85 there have been 8748 reported cases of AIDS[2]. Because PCP occurs in about 60% of these patients[3], it has rapidly become a common disease, seen throughout the general medical wards of many urban hospitals. This change in the epidemiology of PCP has been accompanied by a change in many of its clinical characteristics. For this reason, the review that follows will focus primarily on the clinical presentation and course of PCP in AIDS patients.

EPIDEMIOLOGY

P. carinii is classified as an extracellular protozoan that causes opportunistic infections in immunocompromised hosts. It can be found in three developmental forms - cysts, sporozoites and trophozoites. Cysts, which are found in lung tissue and, less often, respiratory secretions, are usually spherical structures 5 um in diameter that stain best with methanamine silver or toluidine blue O. Within the cysts are found up to eight sporozoites, oval bodies 1-2 um in diameter. The trophozoite forms develop from the excysted sporozoites. They are 2-5 um in diameter, and can be seen with the Gram-Weigert or Giemsa stains[4,5].

P. carinii was first identified in 1942 by VanderMeer in a patient with "interstitial plasma cell pneumonia"[6]. In the following years, epidemics of PCP occurred in malnourished and premature infants in Europe. The first American case was reported in 1956[7]. Between 1956 and 1981 the vast majority of infections have occurred sporadically in patients who are either congenitally, oncologically or iatrogenically immunocompromised. It was not until 1981, that PCP suddenly began appearing in large numbers of previously healthy, immunologically normal men.

The mode of transmission of P. carinii is unclear. Serologic surveys have demonstrated that over 75% of immunologically normal children have acquired antibodies to P. carinii by four years old,[8,9] suggesting reactivation of latent infection in the compromised host. Because infection with P. carinii is almost eclusively limited to the lungs and because the cysts are relatively hardy and can survive in the external environment[10], it is presumed that transmission is via inhalation of cysts. This respiratory mode of transmission has been confirmed in experiments with germfree immunosuppressed rats[15]. It is further supported by reports of PCP epidemics among institutionalized patients that were interrupted by isolation techniques[11], and in families and cohorted cancer patients[12-14]. Thus, despite the notion that disease occurs via reactivation of latent cysts, respiratory isolation should be maintained to protect other immunocompromised patients.

PATHOGENESIS

As mentioned previously, P. carinii is an opportunistic organism of low virulence that causes disease only in the compromised host. This has been well demonstrated in rat models where PCP can be induced in rats that are immunosuppressed with steroids or cyclophosphamide, or compromised by severe malnutrition[16-17]. The precise immunologic deficit that allows reactivation of P. carinii remains unclear and is probably multifactorial.

Among cancer patients, PCP is found most frequently in those with lymphoproliferative disorders[18], with the incidence of disease increasing in relation to the extent of malignancy and the intensity of therapy[19-21]. The disease occurs much less commonly among patients with solid tumors even after they have undergone chemotherapy. This would suggest that it is not malignancy per se that predisposed patients but those malignancies that are most closely involved with immunologic competence, such as in the leukemias and the lymphomas.

The AIDS epidemic may be seen as a tragic human model that supports this notion. While the incidence of PCP in a series of children with primary lymphoproliferative malignancies at St. Jude's Hospital was 5.8%[4], the attack rate in AIDS patients is an astonishing 60%. This can be viewed as a clinical expression of the profoundly disordered immune system that characterizes AIDS patients.

While a detailed discussion of the immunological abnormalities encountered in AIDS is beyond the scope of this review, a brief decription may help to explain both the increased incidence of PCP and the unusual clinical course seen in these patients. Initial reports noted a defect in cell-mediated immunity characterized by greatly decreased numbers of T helper cells and increased numbers of T suppressor cells[22-23]. Since those first papers in 1981, it has been shown that multiple aspects of immunoregulation are affected causing a profound degree of immunoincompetence. Not only is there a quantitative change in T cells and a severe lymphopenia, but those T cells that remain are functionally abnormal as well, unable to respond to antigens and mitogens or provide help to B lymphocytes[24]. B cell immunoglobulin secretion, refractoriness to B cell mitogens, hypergammaglobulinemia and increased immune complexes suggest a polyclonal activation of B lymphocytes[24-26]. In addition to these abnormalities, AIDS patients demonstrate a decreased secretion of lymphokines and gamma interferon[27]. Clearly these patients have a devastating degree of immunodeficiency that combined with malnutrition, makes them extraordinarily vulnerable to _P. carinii_.

PATHOLOGY

Infection with _Pneumocystis_ is virtually always limited to the lung. Rare cases of dissemination to lymph node, liver and spleen have been reported[28-29]. The histopathology has been well reviewed elsewhere[30]. Briefly, there is a range of pathology that begins with the presence of cysts and trophozoites with minimal inflammatory changes. As the cyst population increases, there is a desquamation of alveolar cells. Finally, an intense alveolitis and inflammatory response occurs with an interstitial infiltrate of mononuclear and plasma cells, and clumps of organisms filling the alveoli.

Clinical disease is most frequently seen only as the inflammation and alveolitis develop. It is interesting to note that there are several reports of patients developing PCP as somewhat paradoxically, their steroids were tapered[31].

Conversely, a recent report describes an AIDS patient with PCP whose refractory infection and respiratory failure improved dramatically after adding steroids[32]. These findings suggest that an intact or partially intact inflammatory response is necessary for the expression of overt clinical disease.

CLINICAL MANIFESTATIONS

The clinical characteristics of Pneumocystis pneumonia in the pediatric and oncologic populations have been extensively reviewed elsewhere[19,31,33-34]. The remainder of this discussion will focus on the clinical presentation, course, treatment and prognosis in AIDS patients with PCP. Much of the data and description derive from the experience at a single medical center where over 182 patients with AIDS have been seen and 116 cases of PCP treated between June 1981 and March 1985 (personal communication, Ann Marie O'Brien, RN, Infection Control, St. Vincent's Hospital and Medical Center). The clinical description will be directed towards the initial presentation of patients with PCP who do not have a previous diagnosis of AIDS or opportunistic infections.

Despite the profound immunodeficiency seen in these patients (indeed, perhaps because of it) PCP presents as a subtle and indolent disease. A careful history will frequently elicit two "phases" or "stages" of illness. The patient describes a two to four month history of mild fatigue, malaise, anorexia and weight loss. Often accompanied by low grade fever, sweats and occasionally diarrhea, this frequently is diagnosed as a "viral syndrome". It is followed by four to eight weeks of non-productive cough and subtle but definite dyspnea on exertion. While some patients present with fulminant disease, a detailed history often reveals a long prodrome that was ignored, misunderstood or mistreated. The insidious and subacute nature of this disease in AIDS patients has been well described in several reports [22-23,35-36]. This prolonged course with subtle symptoms contrasts sharply with description of PCP in other immunosuppressed patients[35].

As can be inferred from the above discussion, the key first step towards diagnosis is a high index of suspicion. History taking, in addition to the above, should aim to elicit risk group association (homosexuals, IV drug abusers, hemophiliacs, blood transfusion recipients, prostitutes, Haitians, and sexual partners of high risk individuals), occurrence and frequency of sexually transmitted infections (including Hepatitis B), previous opportunistic infections, and presence of new skin lesions (e.g. Kaposi sarcoma, seborrheic dermatitis, molluscum contagiosum). Of note, is a frequent recent history of herpes zoster in patients who go on to develop AIDS.

A critical step towards early diagnosis is the search for the subtle complaints of minimal hypoxia. Frequently, patients will deny shortness of breath but complain of mildly decreased exercise tolerance or a feeling of breathlessness with exertion. Rarely does a patient complain of shortness of breath at rest unless they are presenting with fulminant disease. However, careful observation during history taking will often reveal that the patient becomes mildly, almost unconsciously, breathless while speaking.

On examination, patients are often found to be cachectic with temporal muscle wasting. They are usually febrile without rigors. Of particular note is the frequent finding of tachycardia out of proportion to the fever or respiratory rate. Lymphadenopathy is often present and oral candidiasis is nearly always found. Fundoscopic examination may reveal cotton-wood spots secondary to P. carinii or chorioretinitis caused by CMV[27,24]. Rales can be heard on pulmonary examination, but are frequently absent. Dermatological evaluation often demonstrates a flakey seborrheic dermatitis of the face and scalp, and occasionally lesions consistent with Kaposi's sarcoma. The remainder of the examination is usually nonspecific although hepatosplenomegaly may be present and a careful neurologic examination may reveal findings suggestive of the subacute encephalitis associated with AIDS[38].

The laboratory data obtained on first presentation is generally non-specific, although, of course, patients with recurrent or fulminant disease will have very abnormal values. They are usually mildly anemic and moderately leukopenic and lymphopenic with counts ranging from 2500-4500 and 300-800 respectively. Occasionally patients will present initially with thrombocytopenia or leukocytosis. The sedimentation rate is almost invariably elevated, frequently over 100 mm/hr. Serum albumin levels are usually decreased in the range of 2.5 to 3 g/dl and liver function tests mildly increased[22,23,25].

Perhaps the most critical laboratory test in the early diagnosis of Pneumocystis pneumonia is the arterial blood gas (ABG). As previously mentioned, patients often present with minimal pulmonary complaints, and respiratory rates of 20-25. ABG on room air usually reveals mild hypoxemia with a pO_2 in the range of 70-80 mm Hg and a slightly abnormal alveolar-arterial gradient. Frequently the pO_2 on room air will be over 90 mm Hg and interpreted as normal[35]. However, a careful evaluation of the pH and pCO_2 is often the key to increased suspicion and early diagnosis. Patients with minimal signs and vague symptoms will almost invariably demonstrate a respiratory alkalosis and mild to moderate hypocarbia with the pH ranging from 7.45-7.50 and the pCO_2 from 25mm Hg to 35 mm Hg. These findings, in the appropriate clinical setting, even with a normal chest x-ray, usually dictate the need for further, aggressive diagnostic evaluation.

The x-ray appearance of PCP can be extremely variable. Classically, patients present with bilateral interstitial infiltrates which have ben variously decribed as a diffuse ground-glass pattern[39], symmetric perihilar pneumonia[40], diffuse reticulo-nodular pattern[23] and hazy perihilar infiltrates which spread to the periphery[5]. Because PCP is a diffuse alveolar process, the infiltrates commonly coalesce and air bronchograms become apparent. As the disease progresses, particularly if respiratory failure develops, extensive bilateral consolidation and even opacification can occur[39,41,42]. Atypically patients may present with a lobal consolidation[43], asymptomatic focal infiltrates[40] isolated nodules[44,23], and rarely, hilar or paratracheal lymphadenopathy[39]. Pleural effusions are almost never found in early disease.

To further complicate the diagnostic picture, patients may often present with a normal chest X-ray[45,22,36]. This has become increasingly more common as the clinical experience and index of suspicion grows and patients are seen and evaluated at earlier stages of disease. The gallium scan has become an important radiographic tool in this situation[45-46]. In the proper clinical setting, and despite a normal chest x-ray, gallium uptake in the lungs should direct the clinician towards an aggressive diagnostic approach in an effort to obtain an early diagnosis (Fig 1-3).

DIAGNOSIS

Commonly, a patient clinically suspected of having PCP is started on therapy pending a definitive diagnosis. Every effort should be made to obtain a tissue diagnosis within 48-72 hours for three major reasons. First and perhaps most importantly, immunocompromised patients are not only vulnerable to many other diseases which can mimic the clinical picture of PCP (e.g. CMV, cryptococcal, toxoplasma and cryptosporidial pneumonitis, Mycobacterium avium, Kaposi's sarcoma, and legionnaires' disease), but are frequently found to have multiple pulmonary processes which would alter therapy[24,31,35,47-49]. Second, after several days of therapy, the organism becomes more difficult to identify and the histological "background" changes. Finally, it is not uncommon for AIDS patients with PCP to enter the hospital with indolent disease and then rapidly deteriorate making diagnostic procedures more difficult and dangerous.

While P. carinii can occasionally be found in sputum, definitive diagnosis usually requires an invasive procedure. Most medical centers seeing large numbers of AIDS patients now routinely perform bronchoscopy with bronchoalveolar lavage and transbronchial biopsy. The risks of pneumothorax and bleeding are minimal and the primary contraindication is severe hypoxia. Rarely, the diagnosis is made by percutaneous needle biopsy of an isolated nodule (Personal communication, Dr. Harry Moussaris, St. Vincent's Hospital). If bronchoscopy fails to yield a diagnosis, and the patient is not responding to appropriate therapy, then an open lung biopsy should be performed.

Diagnostic material should be sent for bacterial, fungal, protozoan, mycobacterial, legionella and viral stains, culture and fluorescent antibody studies. As mentioned above, because PCP is so frequently complicated by other concurent infections, the laboratory evaluation must be comprehensive. The pathology laboratory should receive specimens for histological evaluation to confirm the microbiological diagnosis and to rule out other processes such as Kaposi's sarcoma and non-Hodgkin's lymphoma. In addition to the need for careful coordination among the various physicians, technicians and services, the life threatening nature of these diseases makes it imperative that a diagnosis be made as rapidly as possible.

The laboratory procedures and stains used in the diagnosis of Pneumocystis pneumonia and other opportunistic pathogens has been well reviewed elsewhere[50,51-55]. Table 2 represents a comprehensive protocol on how to handle and process specimens to achieve a detailed diagnostic profile of pulmonary disease in AIDS patients. At our institution, under the direction of Dr. Pearl Ma, the use of touch preparation material and the Hemacolor stain has facilitated the very rapid diagnosis of PCP. Confirmation is then obtained using the various procedures outlined in Tables 1 and 2. While the antibody and antigen aspects of diagnosis continue to be studied, they are not, at present, useful for the accurate diagnosis of acute infection with Pneumocystis carinii.

TREATMENT

Because early diagnosis and treatment appear to improve the outcome, patients are usually started on therapy pending a definitive tissue diagnosis. Trimethoprim-sulfamethoxazole (TMP-SXT) or pentamidine isethionate are the only two available drugs that have been shown to be clearly effective against P. carinii. Since 1978, the first drug of choice has been TMP-SXT, because it was found to be equally effective and less toxic than pentamidine[58]. However, as will be discussed below, this choice

Table 1. Handling of tissue specimens for evaluation of pulmonary disease in AIDS patients.

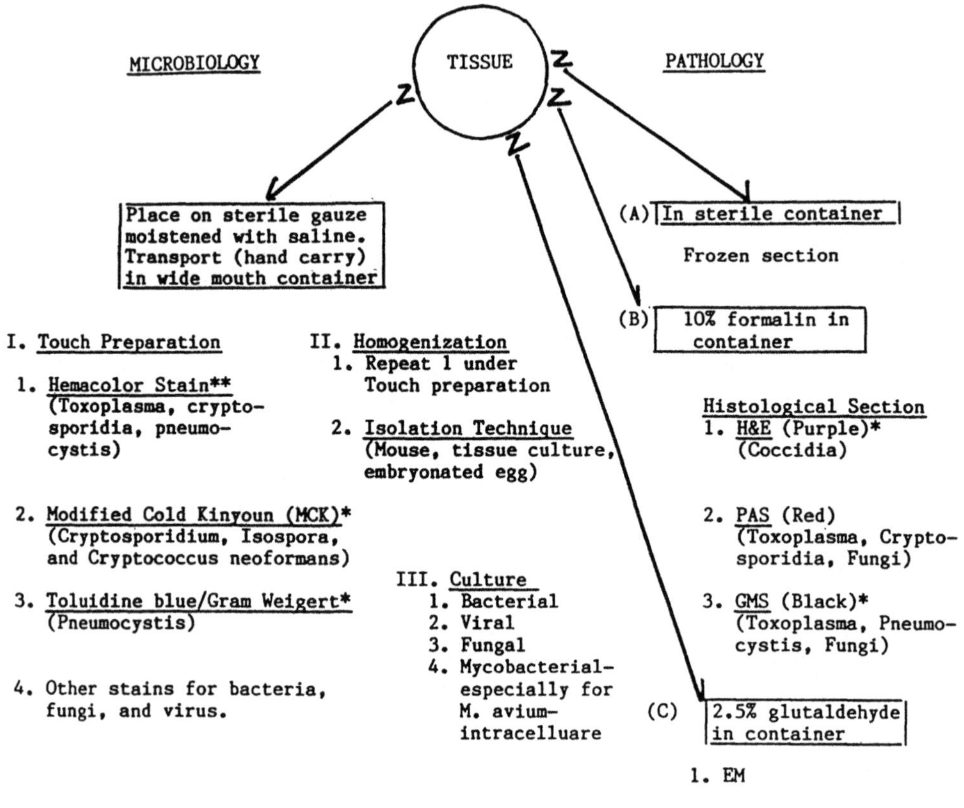

Z indicates procedures to be carried out immediately in the operating room; ** rapid 1 minute staining, preliminary diagnosis; * differential staining confirmation. H&E, Hematoxylin and eosin; PAS, periodic acid-Schiff; GMS, Grocott methenamine silver; EM, electron microscopy. (Adapted from Dr. Pearl Ma, in Microbiology - 1984, Leive, L. and Schlessinger, D. (eds). American Society for Microbiology. Washington, D. C., 1984.)

Table 2. Laboratory diagnosis of pulmonary opportunistic infections in patients with AIDS.

Infection	Clinical Specimens		Identification Profile	
Parasites				
Pneumocystis carinii	Lung biopsy Bronchial lavage		Touched preparation-Hemacolor stain (1 minute) Gram-Weigert's (15 minutes) Toluidine blue (30 minutes)-cyst wall stained Histologic section-H and E foamy cellular reaction Gomori Methenamine Silver-cyst wall black	
Toxoplasma gondii	Lung biopsy		Touch preparation Histologic section-H and E Necrosis-tachyzoites, tissue cyst (100 um) with bradyzoites Mouse inoculation-IP/SC 7 to 14 days (+)	
Cryptosporidiosis, pulmonary	Sputum Lung biopsy		Cryptosporidium oocyst 4-5 um oval/ spherical	Pneumocystis carinii cysts 5-6 um oval spherical
		Giemsa/ Hemacolor	cytoplasm-purple	purple
		GMS	Negative	Black
		Modified Cold Kinyoun (MCK)	acidfast (+) Red	acidfast (-) Green
Fungi				
Candidiasis	Sputum Lung biopsy		Direct smear and culture Conventional procedure	
Cryptococcal pneumonitis	Sputum Lung biopsy		India Ink Culture MCK -reveals capsule distinctively	
Legionaires Disease	Sputum Lung biopsy		DFA IFA Culture	
Viruses				
Disseminated cytomegaloviral infection	Lung biopsy		Tissue-"owl eye" inclusion (Cowdry Type A) single, large eosinophilic intranuclear inclusion surrounded by a "halo" in susceptible cells	
M. tuberculosis M. avium-intracellulare	Lung biopsy Sputum		Acid fast staining Culture Blood culture (for M. avium)	

*H and E = hematoxylin and eosin stain; IFA = indirect fluorescent antibody test;IHA = indirect hemagglutination test; IP = intraperitoneal inoculation; SC = subcutaneous inoculation; GMS = gomori methenamine silver and DFA = direct flourescent antibody test. Adapted from Dr. Pearl Ma, (55).

may not be appropriate for AIDS patients with PCP.

TMP-SXT is given orally or intravenously in doses of 20 mg trimethoprim per kilogram and 100 mg sulfamethoxazole per kg in four divided doses for 14 days. While adequate serum levels and responses can be achieved with oral therapy[47], the drug often causes intolerable gastrointestinal side-effects or patients are simply too ill for oral treatment. Occasionally, it is possible to begin intravenous therapy and after a clear-cut clinical response, switch to oral therapy.

As experience with AIDS patients and the treatment of PCP has grown, two major problems concerning the use of TMP-SXT have become clear: a surprisingly frequent incidence of apparent ineffectiveness and an extremely high level of adverse drug reactions[24,35,47,57]. The first 4-7 days of therapy with this drug are critical. It is during this period that allergic reactions usually occur or treatment failure becomes evident. After excluding those patients who have a toxic drug reaction requiring cessation of therapy, approximately 30% require a change of drug because of advancing disease[47,57]. Clinical response can be assessed by evaluating the patient's respiratory function, temperature, and chest x-ray. The picture however, is often confusing because changes in the chest x-ray often lag behind the clinical improvement, and persistent fever may be secondary to a drug reaction. Perhaps the two most accurate indicators of clinical response are the arterial blood gas and the patient's subjective statements about his sense of well being. A worsening hypoxia with increased hyperventilation may lead rapidly to respiratory failure and should suggest an urgent re-evaluation of therapy. Conversely, a patient who says he feels better, more comfortable and less short of breath, is, despite persistent fever and abnormal chest x-rays, probably responding to therapy.

Unlike other immunodeficient patients with PCP, AIDS patients have an extraordinarily high incidence of adverse reactions to TMP-SXT[35,57]. Approximately 65% of patients demonstrate significant toxicity and about one-half of these are severe enough to require a change in therapy. Between one third and one half of the patients develop fever, rash or leukopenia, while significant thrombocytopenia and hepatitis occur less frequently. These adverse reactions often occur together, greatly complicating the clinical picture. In our experience leukopenia occurs in nearly 100% of patients and is unaffected and not prevented by the use of folinic acid. The fever and rash may sometimes be controlled with antihistamines[58] and antipyretics, and they occasionally resolve spontaneously as therapy continues. While the leukopenia is disturbing, it rarely becomes clinically significant in those patients who successfully complete a full course of treatment. The decision to alter therapy is a difficult one, particularly if other evidence suggests that the disease is responding, and requires careful and frequent clinical evaluation.

Because TMP-SXT is so poorly tolerated and frequently ineffective, pentamidine has become more widely used. It is administered intramuscularly or intravenously as a single daily dose at 4 mg/kg of body weight for 14 days. If pentamidine is given after a TMP-SXT failure, it is still usually continued for an additional 2 weeks. In treating AIDS patients longer courses of either drug are frequently necessary to achieve a complete clinical response, and it is not uncommon for patients to receive four weeks of treatment. It is important to note that there is no clear benefit to combined therapy with both drugs, and that the risk of adverse reactions may be significantly increased[47]. When pentamidine is given as the initial therapy or started after TMP-SXT toxicity, the two drugs appear to be equally effective. However, when pentamidine is used because of TMP-SXT failure, the outcome is poor[47,57].

About 50% of patients experience some form of drug toxicity with pentamidine. Infrequent reactions include rash, leukopenia, thrombocytopenia and fever. The hematologic effects can sometimes be severe and require cessation of therapy. Azotemia and hepatitis can occur more frequently but rarely require a change in treatment.

Until recently, it was recommended that pentamidine be given intramuscularly because of reports of severe hypotension following rapid intravenous administration. However, recent experience with the drug appears to contradict this finding. A survey by the Centers for Disease Control found that hypotension occurred only in patients given IM injections. When the drug was diluted in 100cc. of fluid and administered slowly over one hour there was no effect on blood pressure[60]. Use of the IV route also avoids the development of painful sterile abscesses, a complication seen in approximately 15% of patients receiving intramuscular injections[35,60]. In some patients, perhaps because of cachexia and consequent chemical or mechanical nerve injury, repeated IM injections have resulted in mild to severe peripheral neuropathies (unpublished personal observation). In view of the above, and because the other adverse effects are not related to route of administration, we now give pentamidine intravenously.

Perhaps the most serious and problematic toxicity of pentamidine is its effect on glucose metabolism. About 10% of patients will experience hypoglycemia and in some it may be life threatening and prolonged [35,57,61-63]. The problem usually develops during the second week of therapy though it can occur after the first dose[61]. Hypoglycemia can appear several hours after the dose of medication and is associated with inappropriately high levels of insulin[61-63]. The sustained hypoglycemia that occurs in some patients can be successfully treated with oral or intravenous diazoxide[63]. Paradoxically, some patients, weeks after pentamidine therapy is completed, develop insulin dependent diabetes. These adverse effects can be explained by studies which suggest that pentamidine has a cytolytic effect on the beta-cell, initially causing increased release of insulin followed by destruction and the onset of type I diabetes[61-62]. This serious sequence of events must be anticipated and monitored during and after use of pentamidine.

Because treatment with TMP-SXT and pentamidine is often unsuccessful and carries such a high incidence of toxicity there is a great need for new agents. Diaminodiphenylsulfone (Dapsone) and alpha-Difluormethylornithine (DFMO) are currently undergoing clinical trials. Dapsone, a drug long used in the treatment of leprosy, is being investigated because animal studies have shown it to be effective against P. carinii both as primary therapy and as prophylaxis[64]. DFMO is a new agent which has been used successfully to treat several protozoan infections in both animals and humans[65]. In a preliminary trial, the drug was effective in six AIDS patients with PCP who were intolerant or unresponsive to pentamidine and trimethoprim-sulfamethoxazole[65]. DFMO is presently being more widely studied with promising results and relatively low toxicity.

PROGNOSIS

Pneumocystis carinii pneumonia is a grim disease. Untreated, it has a mortality rate of nearly 100%[5]. With conventional therapy, survival rates for AIDS and non-AIDS patients is 50-60%[35]. However, for AIDS patients these statistics require further scrutiny, as they reflect overall survival of all patients from each episode of acute infection. Our experience has shown that patients who present with PCP as their initial opportunistic infection, without respiratory failure, have survival rates close to 90%. Patients with recurrent infection, concurrent opportunistic infections or Kaposi's sarcoma have much lower survival statistics. Those patients who present in respiratory failure requiring mechanical ventilation have a dismal prognosis, though this appears to be improving. Prior to October 1984, 35 patients with biopsy prove PCP and respiratory failure were admitted to the St. Vincent's Hospital ICU and only two survived. In the following 5 months only 7 patients with PCP required mechanical ventilation and 4 of these survived (personal communication, M. DeVita, M.D., SVH). This dramatic improvement is probably a result of earlier diagnosis and initiation of treatment combined with greater ICU experience in the management of this disease.

Despite apparently adequate therapy, approximately 20% of AIDS patients will have recurrent episodes of PCP[24,35,66]. Based on previous studies, TMP-SXT has been used as prophylaxis against recurrent infection[67-68]. Unfortunately, the high incidence of adverse ractions has occurred even with the small doses used in chemoprophylaxis, limiting this drug's usefulness. Pyrimethamine-sulfadoxine (Fansidar) has been used successfully to prevent recurrent disease, even in patients with prior hypersensitivity reactions to TMP-SXT[66]. However, a recent report from the CDC noted several fatal allergic reactions to Fansidar and cautioned against its use in sulfa sensitive patients[69]. Possibly, DFMO and Dapson may emerge as new prophylactic drugs. However, while early diagnosis, meticulous care and new agents may improve the outcome in P. carinii pneumonia, the ultimate prognosis for patients with the Acquired Immune Deficiency Syndrome remains grave, with a two year mortality rate of nearly 100%[24].

REFERENCES

1. C.D.C., Pneumocystis pneumonia -- Los Angeles, MMWR 30:250-2 (1981).
2. C.D.C., National Surveillance.
3. Jaffe, H.W., Bregman, D.J. and Selik, R.M., Acquired immune deficiency syndrome in the United States, the first 1000 cases, J. Infect. Dis. 148:339-45 (1983).
4. Anderson, D.L., Pneumocystis carinii pneumonia in Fergen, R.D., Cherry, J.D., Textbook of Pediatric Infectious Disease, WB Saunders Co., Philadelphia, 215-222 (1981).
5. Myers, J.D., Pneumocystis carinii pneumonia in Petersdorf, R.G. etc., Harrison's Principles of Internal Medicine. McGraw Hill, New York, 1206-1207 (1983).
6. VanderMeer, G., and Brug, S.L., Infection par pneumocystic chez l'homme et chez les animaux, Ann. Soc. Belge Med. Trop. 22:301 (1942).
7. Dauzier, G., Willis, T., and Barnett, R., Pneumocystis carinii in an infant, Am. J. Clin. Path. 26:787-793 (1956).
8. Meuwissen, H.H. E. Th., Tauber, I., Leeuwenberg, A.D.E.M., et al., Parasitologic and serologic observations of infection with pneumocystis in humans, J. Infect. Dis. 136:43 (1977).
9. Pifer, L.L., Hughes, W.T., Stagno et al., Pneumocystis carinii infection: evidence for high prevalence in normal and immunosuppressed children, Pediatrics 61:35 (1978).

10. Hughes, W.T., Price, R.A., Kim, H. et al., Pneumocystis carinii pneumonitis in children with malignancies, J. Pediat. 82:404-416 (1983).
11. Sheldon, W., Pulmonary Pneumocystis carinii infection, J. Pediat. 61:;780-791 (1962).
12. watnabe, J.M., Chinchinian, J., Weitz, C. et al., Pneumocystis carinii pneumonia in a family, J.A.M.A. 193:685-686 (1965).
13. Brazinsky, J.H., Phillips, J.E., Pneumocystis pneumonia transmission between patients with lymphoma, J.A.M.A. 209:1527-1529 (1969).
14. Singer, C., Armstrong, KD., and Rosen, P.P., Pneumocystis carinii pneumonia. A cluster of eleven cases, Ann. Intern. Med. 82:772-777 (1975).
15. Hughes, W.T., Natural mode of acquisition for de novo infection with Pneumocystis carinii, J. Infect. Dis. 145:842-848 (1982).
16. Frenkel, J.K., Good, J.T., and Schulata, J.A., Latent pneumocystis infections of rats; relapse and chemotherapy, Lab. Invest. 15:1559-1577 (1966).
17. Hughes, W.T., Price, R.A., Sisko, F., et al., Protein-calorie malnutrition; a host determinant for Pneumocystis carinii infection, Am. J. Dis. Child. 128(1):44-52 (1974).
18. Burke, KB.A., and Good, R.A., Pneumocystis carinii infection, Medicine 52:23 (1973).
19. Hughes, W.T., Feldman, S., Aur, R.J. et al., Intensity of immunosuppressive therapy and the incidence of Pneumocystis carinii pneumonitis, Cancer 36(6):2004-2009 (1975).
20. Perera, D.R., Western, K.A., Johnson, H.D., et al., Pneumocystis carinii pneumonia in a hospital for children, epidemiologic aspects, J.A.M.A. 214:1074-1078 (1970).
21. Simone, J.V., Aur, R.J., Hustu, H.O., et al., Acute lymphocytic leukemia in children, Cancer 36:770-774 (1975).
22. Gottlieb, M.S., Scroff, R., Schanker, H.M., Weisman, J.D., Fan, P.T., Wolf, R.A., Saxon, A., Pneumocystis carinii pneumonia and mucosal candidiasis in previously healthy homosexual men, N. Engl. J. Med. 305:1425-31 (1981).
23. Masur, H., Michelis, M.A., Greene, J.B., et al., An outbreak of community-acquired Pneumocystis carinii pneumonia: initial manifestations of cellular immune dysfunction, N. Engl. J. Med. 305:1431-1438 (1981).
24. Fauci, A.S., moderator, Acquired immunodeficiency syndrome: epidemiologic, clinical, immunologic, and therapeutic considerations, Ann. Intern. Med. 100:92-106 (1984).

25. Lane, C.H., Masur, H., Edgar, L.C., Whalen, G., Rook, A.H., Fauci, A.S., Abnormalities of B-cell ctivation and immunoregulation in patients with the acquired immunodeficiency syndrome, N. Engl. J. Med. 309:453-8.
26. Pahwea, S.G., Quilop, M.T.J., Lange, M., Pahwa, R.N., Grieco, M.H., Defective B-lymphocyte function in homosexual men in relation to the acquired immunodeficiency syndrome, Ann. Intern. Med. 101:757-763 (1984).
27. Murray, H.W., Rubin, B.Y., Masur, H., Roberts, R.B., Impaired production of lymphokines and immune (gamma) interferon in the acquired immunodeficiency syndrome, N. Engl. J. Med. 310:883-889 (1984).
28. Henderson, D.W., Humeniuk, V., Meadows, R., et al., Pneumocystis carinii pneumonia with vascular and lymph nodal involvement, Pathology 6(3):235-241.
29. Rahimi, S.A., Disseminated Pneumocystis carinii in thymic alymphoplasia, Arch. Pathol. 97:162-165 (1974).
30. Price, R.A., and Hughes, W.T., Histopathology of Pneumocystis carinii infestation and infection in malignant disease, Hum. Pathol. 5:737-752 (1974).
31. Burke, B.A., and Good, R.A., Pneumocystis carinii infection, Medicine, 52:23-51 (1973).
32. Foltzer, M.A., Hannon, S.E., Kozak, A.J., Pneumocystis pneumonia: response to corticosteroids, J.A.M.A. 253:979 (1985).
33. LeClair, R.A., Pneumocystis carinii and interstitial plasma cell pneumonia, a review, Am. Rev. Resp. Dis. 96:1131-1136 (1967).
34. Walzer, P., Perl, D.P., Krogstad, D.J., et al., Pneumocystis carinii pneumonia in the United States, Ann. Intern. Med. 80:83-93 (1974).
35. Kovacs, et al., Pneumocystis carinii pneumonia: A comparison between patients with the acquired immunodeficiency syndrome and patients with other immunodeficiencies, Ann. Intern. Med. 10:663-671 (1984).
36. Follansbee, S.E., Busch, D.F., Wofsy, C.B., et al., An outbreak of Pneumocystis carinii pneumonia in homosexual men, Ann. Intern. Med. 96:(6 Pt 1):705-713 (1982).
37. Kwok, S., O'Donell, J.J., Wood, I.S., REtinal cotton-wool spots in a patient with Pneumocystis carinii infection, N. Engl. J. Med. 307:184-185 (1982).
38. Snider, W.D., Simpson, D.M., Nielson, S., Gold, J.W.M., Metroka, C.E., Posner, J.B., Neurological complications of acquired immune deficiency syndrome: analysis of 50 patients, Ann. Neurol. 14:403-418 (1983).
39. Gamsu, G., Hecht, S.T., Birnberg, F.A., Coleman, D.L., Golder J.A., Pneumocystis carinii pneumonia in homosexual men, A.J.R. 139:653-658 (1982).

40. McCauley, D.I., Naidich, D.P., Leitman, B.S., Reede, D.L., Lauberstein, L., Radiologic patterns of opportunistic lung infections and Kaposi's sarcoma in homosexual men, A.J.R. 139:653-658 (1982).
41. Doppman, J.L., Geelhoed, G.W. and DeVita, V.T., Atypical radiographic features in Pneumocystis carinii pneumonia. Radiology, 114(1):39-44 (1975).
42. Forest, J.V., Radiographic findings in Pneumocystis carinii pneumonia. Radiology 103:539-544 (1972).
43. Byrd, R.B., Horn, B.R., Infection due to Pneumocystis carinii simulating lobar bacterial pneumonia, Chest. 70:91 (1976).
44. Cross, A.S., Stigbigel, R.T., Pneumocystis carinii pneumonia presenting as a localized nodular densities, N. Engl. J. Med. 291:831 (1984).
45. Levin, M., et al., Pneumocystis pneumonia: Importance of gallium scan for early diagnosis and description of a new immunoperoxidase technique to demonstrate Pneumocystis carinii, Am. Rev. Respir. Dis. 128:182-185 (1983).
46. Turbiner, E.H., Yeh, S.J., Rosen, P.P., Manjlt, S.B., Benua, R.S., Abnormal gallium scintigraphy in Pneumocystis carinii pneumonia with a normal chest radiograph, Radiology 127:437-8 (1978).
47. Haverkos, H.W., Assessment of therapy for Pneumocystis carinii pneumonia, Am. J. Med. 76:501-507.
48. Theolgides, A., Pflueger, O.H., and Kennedy, B.J., Toxoplasmosis and Pneumocystis carinii pneumonia, Minn. Med. 52:737-742 (1969).
49. Ma, P., Villanueva, T.G., Kaufman, D., Gilhooley, J.F., Respiratory Cryptosporidiosis in the Acquired Immune Deficiency Syndrome, J.A.M.A. 252:1298-1301 (1984).
50. Kim, H.K. and Hughes, W.T., Comparison of methods for identification of Pneumocystis carinii in pulmonary aspirates, Am. J. Clin. Path. 60:462-466 (1973).
51. Rosen, P.P., Martini, N., Armstrong, D., Pneumocystis carinii pneumonia: diagnosis by lung biopsy, Am. J. Med. 58:794-802 (1975).
52. Chalvarjian, A.M., Grawe, L.A., A new procedure for the identification of Pneumocystis carinii cysts in tissue sections and smears, J. Clin. Path. 383:-4 (1963).
53. Hughes, W.T., Current status of laboratory diagnosis of Pneumocystis carinii pneumonitis, C.R.C. Crit. Rev. Clin. Lab. Sci. 6(2):145-170 (1975).
54. Ma, P., Laboratory diagnosis of sexually transmitted diseases and opportunistic infections in homosexual men, in Ma, P., Armstrong, D. (eds), The Acquired Immune Deficiency Syndrome and Infections in Homosexual Men, Yorke Medical Books, 149-194 (1984).

56. Hughes, W.T., Feldman, S., Chaudhary, S.C., Ossi, M.G., Cox, F., Sanyal, S.K., Comparison of pentamidine isethionate with trimethoprim-sulfamethoxazole inthe treatment of Pneumocystis carinii pneumonia. J. Pediat. 92:285-92 (1978).
57. Gordon, F.M., Simons, G.L., Wofsy, C.B., Mills, J., Adverse reactions to trimethoprim-sulfamethoxazole in patients with the acquired immunodeficiency syndrome, Ann. Intern. Med. 100:495-499 (1984).
58. Gibbons, R.B., Lindauer, J.A., Successful treatment of Pneumocystis carinii pneumonia with trimethoprim-sulfamethoxazole in hypersensitive AIDS patients, J.A.M.A. 253:1259-1260.
59. Kluge, R.M., Spaulding, C.M., Spain, A.J., Combination of pentamidine and trimethoprim-sulfamethoxazole in the therapy of Pneumocystis carinii pneumonia in rats, Antimicrob Agents Chemother. 13:975-978, (1978).
60. Navin, T.R., Fontaine, R.E., Intravenous versus intramuscular administration of pentamidine, N. Engl. J. Med. 31:1701-2 (1984).
61. Bouchard, P.H., Sai, P., Reach, G., Caubarrere, I., Ganeval, D., Assan, R., Diabetes mellitus following pentamidine-induced hypoglycemia in humans, Diabetes 31:40-5 (1982).
63. Fitzgerald, D.B., Young, I., Pentamidine and hypoglycemia (Letter), Ann. Intern. Med. 99:879 (1973).
64. Hughes, W.T., and Smith, B.L., Diamino-diphenylsulfone (Dapsone): a new drug for Pneumocystis carinii pneumonia (abstract), Pedi. Res. 18:277A.
65. Golden, J.A., Sjoerdsuren, A., Santi, D.V., Pneumocystis carinii pneumonia treated with alpha-difluroomethylornithine, West. Jour. of Med. 141:613-623 (1984).
66. Gottlieb, M.S., Knight, S., Mitsuyasu, R., Weismen, J., Roth, M., Young, L., Prophylaxis of Pneumocystis carinii infection in AIDS with pyrimethamine sulfadoxine, Lancet II:8399 (1984).
67. Hughes, W.T., McNabb, P.C. and Makres, T.D., Efficacy of trimethoprim and sulfamehoxazole in the prevention and treatment of Pneumocystis carinii pneumonitis, Antimicrob Agents Chemother. 5:289-293 (1974).
68. Hughes, W.T., Kuhn, S., Chadhary, S., et al., Successful chemoprophylaxis for Pneumocystis carinii pneumonia, Pediatr. Res. 11:501 (1977).
69. C.D.C. - Adverse reactions to Fansifar and update recommendations for its use in the prevention of malaria, M.M.W.R. 33:713-14 (1985).

LIPOSOME TARGETING TO MACROPHAGES: OPPORTUNITIES FOR TREATMENT OF INFECTIOUS DISEASES

Richard Kirsh and George Poste

Smith Kline and French Laboratories
Philadelphia, PA

INTRODUCTION

The central role played by cells of the mononuclear phagocyte system (MPS) such as alveolar macrophages, hepatic Kupffer cells, splenic and lymph node macrophages, tissue histiocytes and circulating blood monocytes in the complex host reaction to neoplastic and infectious diseases has attracted increasing attention during the past 10 years. This interest stems from the experimental studies illustrating that macrophages when appropriately activated* play a major role in host defense against tumors and infectious microorganisms *in vivo* and also display enhanced tumoricidal and microbicidal activity *in vitro*[1-3]. These observations, coupled with the disappointing results obtained in both clinical and experimental studies with immunologically-specific therapeutic modalities mediated by T and B lymphocytes in cancer immunotherapy has led to a renewed interest in the functions of macrophages and NK cells. Additionally, there is needed a reappraisal of the potential therapeutic benefit of augmenting non-specific host defense mechanisms mediated by mononuclear phagocytes for adjunct therapy of neoplastic and infectious diseases. For this reason, a significant effort is now being undertaken by many laboratories to identify and characterize compounds collectively referred to as biological response modifier agents (BRM) that can augment macrophage-mediated host defenses *in vivo*[1,4].

*The term "activated macrophage" used in this article refers only to those macrophages displaying enhanced microbicidal or tumoricidal activity.

The ability to selectively target drugs to specific cells within the body has been one of the most coveted goals in experimental and clinical therapeutics ever since Paul Ehrlich[5] proposed the use of "bodies which possessed a particular affinity for a certain organ...as carriers by which to bring therapeutic agents to the certain organ." Since that time, a wide variety of macromolecular, particulate and cellular matrices have been proposed for use as drug carrier systems. These include: antibodies, dextrans, plasma proteins, polynucleotides, red blood cells, polymorphonuclear leukocytes, gelatin or albumin microspheres, synthetic polymeric nanoparticles, multiphase microemulsions and liposomes[6-9]. Many of these systems have failed to fulfill their initial promise; however, interest in targetable drug delivery systems remains high.

The current information on the application of liposomes to drug delivery in vivo, with specific reference to the use of liposomes for the delivery of antibiotics and BRM to macrophages in vivo for augmenting non-specific host defenses against infectious diseases will be reviewed. Also discussed is the potential toxic liability of liposomal drug carriers and developmental hurdles that must be overcome to ensure the successful commercialization of a liposome-based drug delivery system.

LIPOSOMES

Liposomes are aqueous dispersions of phospholipids forming closed structures composed of either one (unilamellar) or several (multilamellar) lipid bilayers, each bilayer completely surrounding an internal aqueous space. Their potential value as drug carriers stems from their ability to encapsulate a wide variety of water soluble compounds in their internal aqueous space(s) and also incorporate a variety of lipophilic compounds within the lipid bilayer(s). Furthermore, specific recognition ligands such as monoclonal antibodies or integral membrane proteins can be covalently coupled to the surface of the liposomes to serve as targeting molecules to ensure the interaction of the liposomes with defined molecules on target cells[12].

Although many elegant methods have been devised for the preparation of liposomes[10,11], very few were designed for the specific purpose of using liposomes as a drug delivery system. For this reason, the majority of published work on liposome-mediated drug delivery in vivo focuses primarily on two classes of liposomes: small unilamellar liposomes (SUV) and large multilamellar liposomes (MLV). These classes of liposomes were developed largely as model membrane systems for analyzing the physicochemical properties of lipid bilayers and have been adopted largely without modification for use in drug deliver. As such, more emphasis is now being placed on the design of liposomes as drug carriers.

Selection of the appropriate liposome carrier system for drug delivery *in vivo* will depend on the proposed use. Several of the more important factors to consider are: route of administration; dose; physicochemical properties of the drug; drug entrapment efficiency and retention; liposome size; stability in biological fluids; kinetics of clearance from the circulation if injected i.v.; tissue disposition; and the possibility of adverse effects produced by the liposomes themselves or alterations in drug disposition or pharmacokinetics compared with conventional drug formulations[13].

Liposome Targeting to the Mononuclear Phagocyte System

Targeting of liposomes to any specific cell type *in vivo* requires the completion of several independent steps including: access to the appropriate target cell, selective interaction with the target cell and uptake by the target cell with little or no retention or uptake by non-target cells. Furthermore, the drug must remain associated with the liposomes until it is delivered to the target cell and the liposome-drug complex must not induce unacceptable levels of toxicity.

Numerous studies have shown that the majority of liposomes injected i.v. localize primarily in the liver, spleen, and bone marrow irrespective of liposome size, change or structural class[13,14]. Tissue fractionation and ultrastructural studies have established that liposome retention in these organs is primarily due to uptake by mononuclear phagocytes lining the vascular sinusoids in these organs[15]. In addition to uptake by the fixed phagocytic cells in these organs, liposomes can also be phagocytosed by circulating blood monocytes within the vascular system[15].

In discussing the clearance and tissue disposition of liposomes *in vivo*, it is important to note that a number of seemingly minor technical issues can affect these two features of liposome behavior *in vivo* and thus represent a potential source of experimental variation in studies reported by different laboratories. These factors include: purity of phospholipids; size heterogeneity within liposome preparation; storage conditions; liposome permeability and rate of leakage of encapsulated material; dose (Amount of phospholipid/kg body weight; particles/kg body weight; total surface area of particles administered); the age, weight and sex of inoculated animals; and the exact site of injection. Also, in the case of liposomes injected i.v., the volume of inoculum, the diluent and the rate of administration may also affect the kinetics of liposome clearance from the circulation and their tissue disposition[13].

Although phagocytic Kupffer cells lining hepatic sinusoids represent the major site of liposome accumulation *in vivo*, liposomes can also interact with the liver parenchymal cells (hepatocytes). Small sonicated unilamellar liposomes can be taken up by hepatocytes as intact particles[15,16]. In contrast,uptake of intact liposomes of larger size (e.g., MLV) by hepatocytes, if it occurs, is more limited [15,16]. This is presumed to be due to the inability of larger particles to penetrate the gaps in the endothelium lining hepatic sinusoids (see below). Exchange of phospholipids between large MLV liposomes and hepatocytes has been described[16]. This can occur either via direct phospholipid exchange or via indirect transfer of liposomal lipids to high density lipoproteins (HDL) which, in turn, transfer lipid to hepatocytes. Scherphof and his colleagues have obtained evidence which suggests that lipids from liposomes taken up by phagocytic Kupffer cells in the liver can be transferred subsequently to hepatocytes[16].

The other major sites of liposome retention after i.v. injection are the spleen and the bone marrow[13,14]. Liposome accumulation in the spleen is enhanced under conditions where hepatic uptake of liposomes is eliminated. Splenic retention thus represents "spillover" of liposomes from the liver. Saturation of the ability of the spleen to retain liposome results, in turn, in increased "spillover" of liposomes to the bone marrow. Multiple injections of liposomes can eventually "exhaust" the particle retention capacities of liver, spleen and bone marrow[13,14].

Apart from the reports of uptake of intact small sonicated SUV liposomes by hepatocytes described above, there is no evidence of uptake of i.v. administered liposomes as intact structures by cells other than mononuclear phagocytes of the RES and circulating blood monocytes.

The clearance of liposomes from the circulation and their tissue disposition is analogous to the behavior of other inert particulate materials injected i.v. including: colloidal carbon; latex beads; erythrocytes; immune complexes as well as other particulate drug carriers such as nanoparticles and microspheres.

The localization of liposomes injected i.v. in cells of the mononuclear phagocyte system, though frustrating to investigators who wish to direct liposomes to other cells, offers a potentially powerful method for targeting therapeutic agents to these cells. This type of targeting will be referred to as "passive targeting" since it simply exploits the natural fate of liposomes injected i.v. in being taken up by mononuclear phagocytes.

The central role of the MPS in myriad host defense functions is well documented. In addition to its role in removing "foreign" particulate materials, microorganisms, immune complexes, effete cells, dead cells and cell debris from the circulation, the functional state of the MPS is also important in determining host responses to circulatory shock, trauma, surgery, X-irradiation, tissue ischemia and responses to drugs[17]. Many of the host defense functions performed by the MPS are also discharged by blood monocytes, most notably host defense against pathogenic microorganisms, parasites and tumor cells.

The diverse repertoire of host defense functions performed by mononuclear phagocytes suggests that an efficient method for delivery of BRM agents to these cells to augment host defense reactions might have many potential clinical applications. Liposomes represent such a system, though there is presently no reason to assume that liposomes offer any tangible advantage for this purpose over other particulate drug carriers such as nanoparticles and other synthetic microparticle systems that also localize in the RES and blood monocytes following i.v. injection.

Liposomes as Carriers for Antibiotic Therapy

As mentioned above, mononuclear phagocytes play an important role in the clearance and destruction of pathogenic microorganisms; however, a number of bacteria, fungi, viruses and pathogenic protozoa can also replicate intracellularly within macrophages. Intracellular infections are difficult to manage clinically and are often refractory to conventional chemotherapeutic treatment protocols because of poor drug penetration into cells. Administration of the same agents in association with liposomes offers a potential solution to this problem. Assuming that infected macrophages retain their phagocytic capacity, systemic administration of liposomes containing a drug active against the intracellular pathogen provides a method for efficient drug delivery directly to the site of infection. Such site-specific drug targeting may permit the utilization of lower drug doses relative to the amount of free drug used in traditional therapy and thus reduce the potential for toxic side reactions. The merits of this approach for the chemotherapy of intracellular infections of the MPS has been demonstrated by several investigators[18-24,44].

Opportunistic fungal infections caused by *Candida albicans*, *Aspergillus fumigatus* and *Rhizopus spp.* are a major problem in immunologically compromised patients, particularly in patients with neoplastic diseases, such as leukemia and lymphomas[25-27]. The prospect of improved therapy of systemic mycoses using liposome-encapsulated drugs is clinically very important. The demonstration that liposome-encapsulated amphotericin B shows reduced toxicity with no loss of efficacy in the treatment of candidosis, histoplasmosis and cryptococcosis is a major therapeutic achievement[18,20,21,44]. If these findings prove to be a general feature of liposome-associated antifungal drugs it may be possible to develop therapeutic protocols with other compounds that display potent antifungal activity but were dropped from further development due to excessive host toxicity.

Liposome-encapsulated antifungal drugs might reasonably be expected to be of limited success in treatment of infections with the more common opportunistic fungi, where the organisms grow extracellularly. However, selective delivery of antifungal agents to macrophages may still be therapeutically useful. Phagocytic uptake of fungi by macrophages that contain drug would be expected to enhance intracellular destruction of the phagocytosed organisms. In addition, macrophages that had phagocytosed liposomes-containing drug could conceivably act as a mobile slow-release depot. For example, macrophages that endocytosed liposomes containing antifungal drugs while in the circulation may migrate to the site of infection and release compound locally over a prolonged period.

Liposomes as Carriers for Biological Response Modifiers

Macrophages may be rendered microbicidal and tumoricidal by a wide variety of naturally occurring and synthetic agents[1,4]. Two major classes can be identified: microbial cell wall components and lymphokines; molecules from both classes have attracted considerable interest as potential therapeutic candidates.

Direct activation of macrophages can be induced by the interaction of macrophages with agents such as bacterial endotoxin (lipopolysaccharide; LPS), or cell wall components isolated from *Mycobacteria*, *Corynebacteria* or *Nocardia*[28-31]. Most of these agents are unsuitable for clinical use due to significant toxicity. Furthermore, chemical isolation and detailed characterization of microbial cell wall components responsible for macrophage activation has not yet been accomplished. A notable exception is the water-soluble, low-molecular-weight (MW; 459) synthetic dipeptide, N-acetyl-L-alanyl D-isoglutamine (MDP). This molecule is the minimal structural unit that can replace *Mycobacteria* in complete Freund's adjuvant[32]. MDP has been shown to stimulate a variety of macrophage functions *in vitro*, including bactericidal and tumoricidal activities[32,33]. Unfortunately, MDP, though far less toxic than intact bacteria when administered *in vivo*, is inefficient in activating macrophages *in vivo* due to its extremely rapid clearance. More than 90% of MDP injected i.v. is excreted in the urine within 2 hours[33]. Even when MDP is injected i.v. at very high doses (500 ug), it fails to stimulate significant macrophage-mediated antitumor activity[3].

In contrast to bacterial products that act directly on macrophages, indirect macrophage activation can be achieved by lymphokines, released by antigen- or mitogen-stimulated lymphocytes which interact with specific receptors on the macrophage surface[34]. The specific lymphokines responsible for macrophage activation is termed macrophage activation factor (MAF). Current limitations in the separation technology used in lymphokine isolation and characterization dictate that MAF preparations are essentially crude and therefore vary in both chemical composition and biological activity[3].

The use of lymphokine preparations in vivo to render macrophages tumoricidal has been of limited success[35]. Presumably, systemic lymphokine administration has been unsuccessful due to the short biological half-life of circulating lymphokines which is believed to be due to their rapid binding to serum proteins[36]. A more serious limitation is that only a small fraction of the macrophage population may be susceptible to activation with crude lymphokines[37,38]. Following activation, the tumoricidal phenotype decays rapidly after which the macrophages become refractory to subsequent cycles of lymphokine-mediated activation. Thus, at any time a significant fraction of the total macrophage population may be refractory to activation by MAF.

Effective therapy with macrophage activating agents will therefore require compounds that are not only nontoxic and nonimmunogenic but which are also capable of activating macrophages that are refractory to lymphokine activation.

As mentioned above, considerable attention has been given to liposomes as a potential drug delivery system[8,13,14]. Liposomes are a very efficient system for the delivery of agents to mononuclear phagocytes in vivo. Studies on the disposition of liposomes in vivo indicate that following i.v. injection, liposomes localize predominantly in organs with high reticuloendothelial activity such as liver and spleen and in circulating blood monocytes[15]. This "passive" localization of liposomes in mononuclear phagocytes permits the selective delivery of encapsulated materials to these cells in vivo. In addition to delivery of materials to phagocytic reticuloendothelial cells, encapsulation of materials with liposomes serves several other potentially useful functions. Encapsulation of biologically labile materials will protect them from inactivation or degradation in the circulation. Furthermore, compounds such as MDP, which are rapidly cleared from the body when administered as a "free" unencapsulated compound may show extended retention in vivo when administered within liposomes[3].

The passive localization of i.v. administered liposomes within the macrophages of the MPS can be exploited to selectively deliver BRM agents to these cells to enhance their tumoricidal and/or microbiocidal activity. The systemic administration of liposomes containing either lymphokines or synthetic MDP activates macrophage-mediated tumoricidal activity in vitro and in vivo[3,39]. Furthermore, liposome-mediated immunotherapy is effective in augmenting host defense against metastasis and also effective in eradicating established metastases in several murine tumor models.

Koff et al.[40,41] demonstrated that lymphokines encapsulated within liposomes could activate macrophages to selectively destroy Herpes simplex virus type 2 (HSV-2) infected cells while leaving non-infected cells enhanced. In these studies, liposome-encapsulated lymphokines were shown to be at least one thousand times more efficient than "free" unencapsulated lymphokines in rendering macrophages cytolytic towards HSV-2 infected target cells. Although free lymphokines can activate macrophages to lyse virally infected cells in vitro, the efficacy of free lymphokines in vivo is limited by their short biological half-life. By encapsulating lymphokines within liposomes, these agents are protected from inactivation and/or degradation within the circulation, and can be targeted, albeit passively to macrophages within the reticuloendothelial system, including circulating blood monocytes. Thus, if macrophages can be activated by liposome encapsulated lymphokines or MDP in vivo to destroy virus infected cells, this approach may provide a powerful strategy for treatment of viral infections.

Liposome Toxicity and Complications of Liposome Uptake by Mononuclear Phagocytes

Liposomes prepared from most phospholipids and/or cholesterol are biodegradable and single doses are apparently well tolerated by rodents and dogs over a wide dose range. Less is know, however, about the adverse effect of repeated i.v. injection of liposomes on the MPS and other organs.

Recently, we have begun to evaluate the effects of single and multiple liposome doses on MPS clearance capability with respect to the onset, extent and duration of MPS depression[13]. These experiments demonstrated that after a single dose of MLV liposomes the ability to retain a subsequent liposome dose in the liver, spleen and bone marrow recovers fully within 24 hours. In order to evaluate the influence of repeated doses of liposomes on the clearance of a subsequent test does, mice were injected i.v. with up to 20 injections of MLV liposomes prior to injection of a radiolabeled test dose of homologous liposomes. Animals that received more than 10 doses of MLV liposomes displayed a significantly decreased capacity to retain the subsequent test dose. This depression in RE phagocytic capability was not accompanied by a compensatory increase in liposome retention by non-RES organs.

The onset, extent and duration of impaired RES function is dependent on liposome size, dose, dosage frequency and lipid composition[13]. Mice given multiple doses of liposomes at either 3, 7 or 30 day intervals all display significant differences in their ability to clear a subsequent particle dose, with the extent of suppression being more pronounced with the more aggressive dosing schedules. Liposomal lipid composition also influences the retentive capability of the MPS. Liposomes containing diacetylphosphate or sterylamine induced a more rapid onset and a more severe MPS suppression than liposomes prepared from phosphatidylserine and physophatidylcholine or disteroylphosphatylcholine and cholesterol. In addition to direct functional suppression of the MPS particle clearance pathways, multiple doses of multilamellar liposomes can induce bone marrow hypoplasia with resulting decreases in the number of circulating monocytes and granulocytes[13].

Recent reports of the formation of antibodies to a wide range of phospholipids following i.v. injection of liposomes also emphasize the need for caution before a decision is taken to use a multi-dose liposome regimen in man[42].

Liposome Patents and Commercialization

Widespread application of liposomes as particulate drug carriers in clinical therapeutics will obviously require successful commercialization. As with all potential pharmaceutical products, the decision to embark on the high risk, lengthy and expensive development process necessitates not only a clear definition of the scientific and technical merits of the proposed drug design, but a careful examination of both the medical need and the economic demands of product development. The use of drug carriers offers several unique advantages to the pharmaceutical industry. For example, a patent on a novel drug-carrier will extend patent protection to the drug-carrier complex. Assuming that there is a therapeutic advantage to the carrier-associated drug, this provides a powerful strategic approach to counteract generic drug competition. Furthermore, if the drug carrier is suitable for use with several classes of drugs, the expense of carrier development can be diffused.

The potential therapeutic advantages of a liposome-based drug delivery system have been the subject of numerous scientific reports and need not be discussed further. However, the technological and economic feasibility of commercial development of liposomes for use as drug carriers is far from certain. In order to be successful within the foreseeable future, liposome production must be adapted to convenient cost-effective, large-scale preparative methods that will not require extensive process development or a substantial capital investment in ultraspecialized instrumentation. Furthermore, the manufacturing process must be carried out under conditions acceptable to the regulatory agencies. The final product must be homogeneous, have at least a 12-18 month shelf-life and offer maximum convenience to the medical community.

Additional uncertainties arise when one considers that the response of the regulatory agencies that govern the manufacturing and marketing of pharmaceutical products to liposomes or other particulate carrier vehicles has largely gone untested. Although there are no clear precedents, the response of the Food and Drug Administration (FDA) in the U.S. to both pro-drugs and implantable controlled-release polymeric matrices suggests that liposome-associated drugs will be treated as new chemical entities (NCE) and be required to undergo the full range of toxicologic, metabolic and pharmaceutic evaluations required for approval of any new drug administered to patients[43].

Although the demands of solving the scientific, technical and economic problems associated with liposome production seem formidable, there has been extensive U.S. and international patent activity concerning the utilization and production of liposome-mediated drug delivery systems. However, with few exceptions, these patents do not address the methodological problems associated with the large-scale preparation of pharmaceutically-acceptable liposomes. Furthermore, the technical and economic demands of preparing large batches of ultrapure synthetic phospholipids for use in liposome preparation do not appear to be fully appreciated. For example, the FDA guidelines for evaluation of NCE mandate that if a two year toxicology study in dogs is required, this study must use the same batch of carrier-associated drug used in phase II/III clinical trials. Assuming that experimental studies indicate that the effective dose of liposomes required to elicit biological activity is 5 mg phospholipid/mouse,then the total amount of phospholipid required for a complete metabolic and toxicologic profile of the drug carrier system in rats and dogs and a thorough physiochemical characterization of the final liposome formulation to be administered to patients in phases I, II and III clinical studies up to launch of the new liposome-associated drug into the market will require several hundred kilograms of pure phospholipid for each drug tested. Economic considerations such as this clearly suggest that other particulate microcarrier systems such as multiphase emulsions and biodegradable polymeric nanoparticles, which share many of the advantageous properties of liposomes, deserve careful evaluation. Prevailing commercial factors currently favor these alternative drug carriers because they can be produced as pharmaceutically acceptable formulations at far less cost than liposomes using existing equipment and manufacturing processes universally available within the pharmaceutical industry.

Although the demands of solving the scientific and technical problems associated with liposome development are substantial, the extraordinary rate of scientific achievement in both biology and pharmaceutics greatly enhances the prospect of success with at least several aspects of liposome-mediated drug delivery. The next few years will be crucial in determining whether the commercial development of liposomes is feasible or whether they will join the ranks of other drug carrier designs that have failed to fulfill their initial promise.

REFERENCES

1. Pick, E. (ed.), Lymphokines, Vol. 3, Academic Press, NY, (1981).
2. Poste, G., and Fidler, I.J., The pathogenesis of cancer metastasis, Nature, 283:139-146, (1980).
3. Fidler, I.J., and Poste, G., Macrophase-mediated destruction of malignant tumor cells and new strategies for the therapy of metastatic disease, Springer Semin. Immunopathol., 5:161-174, (1982).
4. Chirigos, M.A., Mitchell, M., Mastrangelo, M.J., Krim, M. (Eds.), Modulation of Cellular Immunity in Cancer by Immune Modifiers, Raven Press, NY, (1981).
5. Ehrlich, P., Collected Studies on Immunity, Reprinted, Wiley, NY, Vol. 2, pp. 442-447, (1906).
6. Gregoriadis, G., Sr., and Trouet, A. (Eds.), Targeting of Drugs, Plenum Press, NY, (1982).
7. Bruck, S.D. (Ed.), Controlled Drug Delivery, CRC, Boca Raton, (1982).
8. Gregoriadis, G., and Allison, A.C. (Eds.), Liposomes in Biological Systems, Wiley Interscience, NY, (1980).
9. Poste, G., and Kirsh, R., Site-specific (targeted) drug delivery in cancer therapy, Biotechnology, 1:869-878, (1983).
10. Szoka, F., and Papahadjopoulos, D., Liposomes. Preparation and characterization, in Liposomes: From Physical Structure to Therapeutic Applications, C. G. Knight (Ed.), Elsevier, Amsterdam, pp. 51-82, (1981).
11. Hauser, H., Methods of preparation of lipid vesicles: assessment of their suitability for drug encapsulation, Trends Pharm. Sci., 3:274-277, (1982).

12. Leserman, L.D., Machy, P., Devaux, C., and Barbet, J., Antibody-bearing liposomes: targeting in vivo, Biol. Cell, 47:111-116, (1983).
13. Poste, G., Liposome targeting in vivo: problems and opportunities, Biol. Cell, 47:19-30, (1983).
14. Poste, G., Kirsh, R., and Koestler, T., The challenge of liposome targeting in vivo, in Liposome Technology, G. Gregoriadis (Ed.), CRC Press, Boca Raton, FLA, pp. 1-28, (1983).
15. Poste, G., Kirsh, R., Fogler, W.E., and Fidler, I.J., Analysis of the fate of systemically administered liposomes and implications for their use in drug delivery, Cancer Res., 42:1412-1422, (1982).
16. Scherphof, G.L., Interaction of liposomes with biological fluids and fate of liposomes in vivo, in Liposome Methodology, L.D. Leserman and J. Barbet (Eds.), pp. 79-92, Inserm, Paris, (1982).
17. Altura, B.M., Reticuloendothelial cells and host defense.
18. Taylor, R.L., Williams, D.M., Craven, P.C., Graybill, J.R., Drutz, D.J., and Magee, W.E., Amphotericin B in liposomes; a novel therapy for histoplasmosis, Am. Rev. Respir. Dis 125:610-611 (1982).
19. New, R.R.C., Chance, M.L., and Heath, S., The treatment of experimental cutaneous leishmaniasis with liposome-entrapped Pentostam, Parasitol. 83:519-527 (1981).
20. Lopez-Berestein, G., Mehta, R., Hopfer, R.L., Mills, K., Kasi, L., Mehta, K., Fainstein, V., Luna, M. Hersh, E.M., and Juliano, R., Treatment and prophylaxis of disseminated infection due to Candida albicans in mice with liposomne-encapsulated amphotericin B, J. Infect. Dis. 5:939-945 (1983).
21. Graybill, J.R., Craven, P.C., Taylor, R.L., Williams, D.M., and Magee, W.E., KTreatment of murine cryptococcosis with liposome associated amphotericin B, J. Infect. Dis. 145: 748-751 (1982).
22. Fountain, M.W., Dees, C., and Schultz, R.D., Enhanced intracellular killing of Staphylococcus aureus by canine monocytes treted with liposome containing amikacin, gentamicin, kanamycin, and tobramycin, Current Microbiol. 6:373-376 (1981).
23. Alving, C.R., and Steck, E.A., The use of liposome-encapsulated drugs in leishmaniasis, Trends Biochem. Sci. 4:N175-177 (1979).
24. Desiderio, J.V., and Campbell, S.G., Liposome-encapsulated cephalothin in the treatment of experimental murine salmonellosis, RES: Journal of the Reticuloendothelial Society 34:279-287 (1983).

25. Bodey, G.P., Fungal infections complicating acute leukemia, J. Chron. Dis. 19:667 (1966).
26. Degregorio, M.W., Lee, W.M.F., Linker, C.A., Jacobs, R.A., and Ries, C.A., Fungal infections in patients with acute leukemia, Am. J. Med. 73:543-548 (1982).
27. Louria, D.B., and Sen, P., Fungal infections with a particular focus on the compromised host, Del. Med. J. 54:11-19 (1982).
28. Alexander, P., and Evans, R., Endotoxin and double stranded RNA render macrophages cytotoxic, Nature New Biology 232:76-78 (1971).
29. Cleveland, R.P., Meltzer, M.S., and Zbar, B., Tumor cytotoxicity in vitro by macrophages from mice infected with Mycobacterium bovis strain BCG, J. Nat. Cancer Inst. 52:1887-1894 (1974).
30. Scott, M.T., In vivo cortisone sensitivity of nonspecific antitumor activity of Corynebacteria parvum activated mouse peritoneal macrophages, J. Nat. Cancer Inst. 54:789-792 (1975).
31. Sone, S., and Fidler, I.J., In situ activation of tumoricidal properties in rat alveolar macrophages and rejection of experimental lung metastases by intravenous injections of Nocardia rubra cell wall skeleton, Cancer Immunol. Immunother. 12:203-209 (1982).
32. Lederer, E., Synthetic immunostimulants derived from the bacterial cell wall, J. Med. Chem. 23:819-825 (1980).
33. Parant, M., Parant, F., Chedid, L., Yapo, A., Petit, J.F., and Lederer, L., Fate of the synthetic immunoadjuvant, muramyl dipeptide (^{14}C-labelled) in the mouse, Int. J. Immunopharmacol 1:35-41 (1979).
34. Poste, G., Kirsh, R., and Fidler, I.J., Cell surface receptors for lymphokines, Cell Immunol 44:72-88 (1979).
35. Papermaster, B.W., Holterman, O.A., and Klein, E., Preliminary observations on tumor regressions induced by local administration of a lymphoid cell culture supernatant fraction in patients with cutaneous metastatic lesions, Clin. Immunol. Immunopathol. 5:31 35 (1976).
36. Fidler, I.J., and Raz, A., The induction of tumoricidal capacities in mouse and rat macrophages by lymphokines, in Pick, E. (Ed.), Lymphokines, Vol. 3, Academic Press, New York, pp. 345-364 (1981).
37. Poste, G., and Kirsh, R., Rapid decay of tumoricidal activity and loss of responsiveness to lymphokines in inflammatory macrophages, Cancer Res. 39:2582-2590 (1979).
38. Poste, G., The tumoricidal properties of inflammatory tissue macrophages and multinucleate giant cells, Am. J. Pathol 96:595-608 (1979).

39. Poste, G., and Fidler, I.J., Active non-specific immunotherapy of lung metastases by macrophage activating agents encapsulated in liposome, in Optimization of Drug Delivery, A. Benzon, Symposium No. 17, H. Bundgaard, A. Hansen, and H. Kofod (Eds.), Bundgaard, Copenhage, pp. 48-429 (1982).
40. Koff, W.C., Showalter, S.D., Seniff, D.A., and Hampar, B., Lysis of Herpesvirus-infected cells by macrophages activated with free or liposome-encapsulated lymphokine produced by a murine T cell hybridoma, Infection and Immunity 42:1067-1072 (1983).
41. Koff, W.C., Fidler, I.J., Showalter, S.D., Chakrabarty, M.K., Hampar, B., Ceccorulli, L.M., and Kleinerman, E.S., Human monocytes activated by immunomodulators in liposomes lyse herpesvirus-infected but not normal cells, Science 224:1007-1009 (1984).
42. Alving, C.R., and Richards, R.L., Immunological aspects of liposomes, in The Liposomes, M. Ostro, ed., M. Dekker, New York (In Press) (1983).
43. Federal Register, Food and Drug Administration, Proposed new drug, antibiotic and biologic drug product regulations, 48:26720-749 (June 9, 1983) (1983).
44. Juliano, R.L., Lopez-Berenstein, G., Mehta, R., Hopfer, R., Mehta, K., and Kasi, L., Pharmacokinetic and therapeutic consequences of liposomal drug delivery: fluorodeoxyuridine and amphotericin B as examples, Biol. Cell 47: 39-46 (1983).

BIOLOGICALS AND OTHER BIOLOGICAL RESPONSE MODIFIERS:

PRECLINICAL AND CLINICAL ASSESSMENT IN CANCER TREATMENT

Robert K. Oldham
Biological Response Modifiers Program
National Cancer Instiute-Frederick Cancer Research
Facility, Frederick, Maryland

INTRODUCTION

The investigation of nonspecific immunomodulators as well as the prospect for large numbers of genetically engineered biologicals makes the need for predictive preclinical assays of biological activity and efficacy apparent. In vitro assays of biological activity (bioassays) are generally used to define and quantitate biological activity. Subsequently, enzyme-linked immunosorbent assays, radioimmunoassays, or other methods of determining the number of molecules available allows for the more precise determination of levels of these biologicals. Finally, there is the need to assess the in vivo activity of these materials in preclinical models to develop predictive assays for clinical efficacy and provide information useful in the rational design of clinical trials.

The strategy and design of the Biological Response Modifiers Program (BRMP) preclinical screen and preliminary results with several immunomodulators assessed in this screening program have been reported[1-6]. The evaluation of biologicals such as interferon and the interleukins has been initiated in this screening process. There is often the complicating problem of species specificity as not all lymphokines/cytokines of human origin are active in rodent systems. For example, the naturally occurring human interferons (alpha, beta and gamma) have little activity on rodent cells, making their preclinical assessment difficult. For those biologicals such as interleukin-2 (IL-2) which do have activity on rodent cells, this preclinical system may be of more value.

While lymphokines and cytokines have activity on host biological responses, they may also have some direct activity on tumor cells. This is best exemplified by the direct antiproliferative activity of the interferons. By contrast, monoclonal antibodies are the prototypic substances to be evaluated for specific, direct antitumor activity. Monoclonal antibodies can be designed to act as immunomodulators and affect various components of the immune system, but their early evaluation has centered on their use as specific targeting agents in cancer treatment[7]. A series of studies utilizing an antimelanoma monoclonal antibody[8] or antibody to normal T cells and certain human leukemias and lymphomas[9] have been initiated. It is apparent from these studies that monoclonal antibody can be given intravenously and can be expected, if given in sufficient amounts and in appropriate schedules, to reach the tumor cells variously distributed in the patient. Preliminary results, utilizing the monoclonal antibodies in clinical trials, will be descibed.

PRECLINICAL TESTING PROGRAM

The BRMP preclinical screening system for the assessment of biologicals and biological response modifiers was designed to specifically evaluate the effects of these agents _in vitro_ and _in vivo_ on T and B cells, macrophages, and NK cells. As is illustrated in Table 1, the common track screen is designed to evaluate the effects of these agents on the various cellular and humoral components of the immune response. In addition, specific tracks are being considered to allow for the evaluation of agents and approaches which have more selective targets[1]. More than fifteen compounds have been evaluated in the screening program and as is illustrated in Table 2, immunomodulators have selective activities on certain elements of the immune response. For example, the thymosins, an extract of calf thymus polypeptides, have been most active in T-cell assays but do not enhance NK or macrophage activity, whereas MVE-2 (maleic anhydride-divinyl ether) was more stimulatory for NK cells and macrophages. By contrast, MVE-2 stimulated macrophags and enhanced NK cell activity when given i.v. but did not enhance NK activity when added _in vitro_. This may be explained by MVE-2-stimulated interferon release from macrophages which secondarily activates NK cells _in vivo_. Poly ICLC (Poly inosine-polycysteine) was quite efficacious in stimulating macrophages and NK cells both _in vitro_ and _in vivo_, whereas Nor-muramyldipeptide (N-MDP) was selective for T cells and macrophages but had little stimulatory effect on NK cells. These data illustrate that immunomodulators may selectively effect cetain components of the immune system and some may function _in vitro_ but have little activity _in vivo_. By contrast, others may be effective _in vivo_ but have little activity _in vitro_, particularly when they undergo metabolic activation or alteration.

Table 1. Preclinical Screening of Biological Response Modifiers

Progression	Macrophages	NK Cells	T Cells	B Cells
In vitro activation–in vitro testing	In vitro activation for 24-hr, 72-hr cytotoxicity assay of [^{125}I]IUdR tumor cells and 18-hr [^{111}In] tumor cells	In vitro activation for 24-hr, 4-hr cytotoxicity assay α[^{51}Cr]-YAC	MLR allogeneic MLTR-CMC allogeneic	
In vivo activation–in vitro testing	Inject BRM i.v.; harvest AM and test for tumoricidal activity	Inject BRM i.v.; measure NK activity in vitro IF stimulation	Immunization αTSTA CTL	Stimulation of specific antibody production
In vitro activation–in vivo testing		Prevention of metastasis in 3-wk-old mice (fibrosarcoma)	Immunization αTSTA, s.c. challenge Alteration of tumor growth in UV-irradiated mice after immunization	
Mechanism	Kinetics of activation Induction of hyporesponsiveness	Kinetics of activation Induction of hyporesponsiveness		

Table 2. BRMP Screening Summary

Assay of Immunomodulation	F5[1]	MVE-2[2]	Poly[3] ICLC	Nor-[4] MDP
T-cell blastogenesis	+	-	-	+
Allogeneic MLR stimulation	+	-	-	+
Allogenic MLTR-CMC activation	+	-	-	+
Syngeneic MLTR-CMC activation	+	NT	NT	NT
Immunoadjuvant for specific CTL	+	+	+	+
Immunoadjuvant for tumor challenge	+	+	+	+
In vitro NK cell activiation	-	+	+	-
In vivo NK cell activation	-	-	+	-
In vivo NK cell immunoprophylaxis	-	+	+	-
In vitro macrophage activation	-	+	+	+
In vivo macrophage activation	-	+	+	+
Interferon stimulation	-	+	+	NT

1 Thymosin F5; is an extract of calf thymus polypeptides provided by Hoffmann La Roche, Inc., Nutley, New Jersey. The optimal dose was 12.5 mg/Kg.

2 MVE-2; maleic anhydride-divinyl either, was obtained from Dr. Richard Carreno, Adria Laboratories , Columbus, Ohio. The optimal therapeutic dose was 25 mg/Kg.

3 Poly ICLC; poly inosine-polycysteine stabilized with poly L-lysine and carbozymethyl cellulose was provided by Dr. Hilton Levy, National Institute of Allergy and Infectious Diseases, Frederick, Maryland. Optimal dose was 0.5 mg/Kg.

4 Nor-MDP; Nor-muramyl dipeptide is an analogue of MDP, which is the minimally active subunit from BCG, obtained from Ciba-Geigy, Summit, New Jersey. It had an optimal therapeutic dose of 75 mg/Kg.

5 NT -- Not tested

After the preliminary *in vitro* and *in vivo* testing for immunomodulatory activity, the *in vivo* anti-tumor activity of these compounds was evaluated. Reliance was on those transplantation models which emphasize the evaluation of metastasis and on models of primary tumors utilizing UV light and nitrosomethylurea for tumor induction (Table 3). This emphasis on metastasis and on primary tumors as oposed to standard transplantable laboratory tumors was selected in anticipation that these preclinical models will be more predictive for clinical activity[1].

As is shown in Table 4, several immunomodulators have activity in the inhibition of experimental and spontaneous metastasis. In determining non-specific immunoprophylaxis, the BMR was injected i.v., 48 hours prior to i.v. injection of 50,000 syngenic tumor cells (UV-2237 mm). The mice were necropsied 25 days following tumor challenge and the extent of pulmonary tumor burden quantitated. For specific immunoprophylaxis, the mice were immunized with a suboptimal tumor vaccine consisting of 10^6 irradiated tumor cells obtained by the collagenase-DNAase dissociation of subcutaneous tumors. The BRM was either injected alone or admixed with the tumor vaccine to test its adjuvant activity. Tumor challenge was 10 days following vaccination and consisted of the footpad injection of 10^5 tumor cells. Tumor

Table 3. Preclinical Screening of Biological Response Modifiers: Tumor Therapy Models

Treatment of metastases	Treatment of autochtonous tumors
1. Experimental metasteses	1. UV-induced skin tumors
(survival)	a. Intralesional
(lung colony counts)	b. Twice weekly i.v. for 3 wk
2. Spontaneous metastases	2. NMU-induced mammary tumors
(12 wk)	Twice weekly i.v. for 3 wk
(lung colony counts)	
3. Lifetime survival after experimental and spontaneous metastasis	

Table 4. Comparison of BRM Induced Immunotherapy

	MVE-2[5]	OK-432[6]	Poly ICLC[7]	MTP-PE[8]	A/D BgL[9] IFN	Thymosin F5[10]	Lentanin[11]	NED-137[12]	Nor-[13] MDP
Non-specific immunoprophylaxis[1]	Pos.	Pos.	Pos.	STA[14]	Pos.	Neg.	Neg.	Neg.	Neg.
Specific immunoprophylaxis[2]	Pos.	Pos.	Pos.	Pos.	Pos.	Pos.	STA	Neg.	Pos.
Immunotherapy of experimental metastases[3]	Prolongation of survival	STA	Pos.	Pos.	Pos.	Pos.	STA	Neg.	Pos.
Immunotherapy of spontaneous metastases[4]	Neg.	Neg.	Pos.	Pos.	STA	Pos.	Neg.	Neg.	Pos.

growth and volume was determined weekly. For determination of the immunotherapy of experimental metastases, the mice were injected i.v. with 5 x 10^4 B16-B1-6 tumor cells and 72 hours later therapy was initiated (twice weekly injecting of the BMR for 4 weeks. For measuring spontaneous metastases the B16 cells were injected into the footpad and the limb was resected when the tumor reached an average diameter of 1 cm. Therapy was initiated 72 hours later. Surviving mice wer necropsied 4 weeks after the death of the last saline control to confirm their tumor-free status. The BMR substances included OK-432, a penicillin killed-lyophilized peparation of a virulent strain of group A Streptococcus pyogenes; MTP-PE, muramyl tripeptide-phosphatidyl ethanolamine was incorporated into liposomes; A/D Byl II IFN, a hybrid recombinant interferon; and lentinan, an aqueous extract from the Lentinus edodes mushroom. In addition, evidence is available for the inhibition of autochthonous tumor growth by thymosin fraction 5 and by poly ICLC (Table 5).

Table 5. Therapy of NMU-Induced Mammary Tumors

	Saline	Poly ICLC	Thymosin F5
Mean tumor size at initiation of therapy (cm^3)	0.86 ± 0.97	1.14 ± 1.1	1.29 ± 1.4
Mean tumor size at evaluation (cm^3)	12.11 ± 18.64	5.13 ± 5.69	8.26 ± 1.3
Percent tumor free at evaluation	0%	30%	15%
Percent of animals with multiple tumors	85%	45%	70%
Percent survival at evaluation	90%	95%	90%
Mean time since initiation of therapy (wks)	10.5 ± 2.3	10.5 ± 1.9	10.6 ± 2.0

A single dose of N-nitroso-N-methylurea (50 mg/Kg) was administered intravenously to 50-day old female Sprague Dawley rats. BRM therapy was initiated when the first lesion was noted and consisted of twice a week injection of the agent for four weeks. The BRMs included Poly ICLC at 0.75 mg/Kg and thymosin F5 at 5 mg/Kg with saline controls. Tumor diameters were assessed twice a week and their volume calculated using the formula for a spheroid. The occurrence of satellite tumors is noted and reported as multiple tumors. (N = 20)

These results are encouraging but they also illustrate the complexity of these preclinical tests. The ultimate assessment of the screening program requires the translation of multiple immunomodulating agents into clinical trials to determine whether or not these assays are truly predictive for clinical activity in man. Limited correlations are curently possible for MVE-2, the thymosins, the interferons and may soon be possible for the interleukins.

LYMPHOKINES AND CYTOKINES

Mammalian cells produce a large number of lymphokines and cytokines in response to various stimuli. Cells may produce one or many biologicals when properly induced and these biologicals may each have a complex series of actions on the individual's biological responses. The macrophage is a virtual factory for the production of biologically active factors. Some lymphokines and cytokines appear to be restricted by the major histocompatibility complex (MHC) and these may be characterized as specific or nonspecific. The majority of lymphokines and cytokines are not known to be restricted by the MHC and are not antigen specific. There are over a hundred such substances which have been described by name based on observed biological activity. These substances can be isolated from the products of normal cells, normal cell lines derived from normal tissues, or tumor-derived cell lines. The actual number of lymphokines and cytokines remains to be defined by careful genetic analysis and this will be possible through the production of purified genetically engineered biologicals. A substantial number of these biologicals will soon be cloned and available in sufficient quantities for preclinical and clinical evaluation. This probability makes even more apparent the need for predictive assays of clinical efficacy so resources can be directed toward those biologicals that are most likely to be active in clinical trials. Obviously, the use of these biologicals in therapeutics is not restricted to the cancer therapy, as many of these agents and approaches may be quite useful for autoimmune, inflammatory, and even infectious disorders.

ALPHA INTERFERON

Interferon, as a prototypic biological molecule, has proven very useful in advanceing our understanding of biologicals. Various interferons have greatly different biological effects and the interferons can be active as anticancer agents indirectly through the immune system and by direct effects on the tumor cell[10,11].

The principles of Phase I clinical trials have been

delineating during the development of chemotherapy[12] and have been extended to the phase I testing of biologicals[13]. Phase I clinical trials with alpha-interferons have delineated certain toxocologic and biologic effects in man. While it is recognized that these phase I trials are not designed to measure therapeutic efficacy, approximately 10% of the patients demonstrated an objective antitumor response, most of which fell into selected disease categories such as lymphoma, myeloma, Kaposi's sarcoma, melanoma, renal cancer, and breast cancer[12]. By contrast, very few responses have been seen in patients with the more common malignancies of colon, lung, and the lower genitourinary system. Considerable side effects were asociated with the administration of alpha interferon including fever, chills, headache, fatigue, anorexia, hepatic and haematologic depression, CNS effects and weight loss. Selected phase II data, subdivided into the general categories of alpha-Cantell, alpha-lymphoblastoid, and alpha-recombinant, are summarized in Table 6.

Table 6. Alpha-Interferon Phase II Studies

Tumor Type	Interferon	Dose	CR & PR
Lung	α-Cantell	3 mu/d x 5	1/37
Breast	α-Cantell	3-9 mu daily	7/17
Breast	α_2-Recombinant	50/mu/m^2 3x/wk	0/17
Breast	α-Cantell	3 mu daily	5/23
Colon	α-Cantell	3 mu/d x 5	0/19
Colon	α_2-Recombinant	5 mu tiw	1/18
Colon	α-Lymphoblastoid	3 mu/m^2 3x/wk	0/19
Carcinoid	α-Cantell	3-6 mu/daily	6/9
Ovary	α-Cantell	1-6 mu daily	1/15
Renal	α-Cantell	3 mu daily	5/19
Renal	α_2-Recombinant	50 mu tiw	2/19
Renal	α_2-Recombinant	2 mu/m^2 daily	0/8
Renal	α_2-Recombinant	20 mu/m^2 daily	2/8
Melanoma	α-Lymphoblastoid	2.5 mu/m^2 daily	1/17
Melanoma	α_2-Recombinant	50 mu/m^2 3x/wk	7/31
Melanoma	α-Cantell	3-9 mu daily	6/10
Lymphoma	α_2-Recombinant	50 mu/m^2 3x/wk	26/42
Lymphoma	α-Cantell	3-9 mu daily	6/11
Kaposi	α_2-Recombinant	36-54 mu daily	14/34
Hairy Cell Leukemia	α-Cantell	3 mu daily	10/11
CML	α-Cantell	9-15 mu daily	22/25

Summarized from and referenced in (18).

BETA INTERFERON

Beta-interferon produced by cultured fibroblasts under appropriate stimulation has been used in clinical trials over the past several years. This "natural" beta-interferon has been somewhat difficult to purify and, given the low purity of preparations available, doses up to 10 million units per m^2 have been tolerated with side effects similar to those seen with the alpha-interferons. In these early phase studies it was noted that beta-interferon was inactivated rapidly in muscle but when given i.v. had effects similar to those seen with alpha - interferon. The need for i.v. administration and the short half-life, as well as the lower doses that were tolerated by patients, characterized these natural beta-interferons. Subsequent studies with more purified preparations of natural beta-interferon as well as data with recombinant beta-interferon would indicate that these interferons may be tolerated in doses up to several hundred million units per m^2 and have clinical effects similar to those seen with recombinant alpha-interferons. Trials with recombinant beta-interferon will further define its biological effects and antitumor activity.

GAMMA INTERFERON

Extensive testing of the alpha-interferons and the early testing for the beta-interferons have emphasized their antiviral activity and their potential antiproliferative activity in man. Both of these interferons also have immunomodulatory effects and these effects are analyzed concomitantly. However, preclinical studies would seem to indicate that gamma-interferon is a more diverse and powerful immunomodulator than alpha- or beta - interferon and there are indications that it may be responsible for some of the biological activities previously ascribed to other lymphokines and cytokines[14-17]. Recombinant gamma-interferon is currently in clinical trials and it will be of great interest to detrmine which biological responses are reproducibly altered by its administration. Information from previous trials of partially purified natural gamma-interferon would suggest that the i.v. route is necessary to achieve antiviral serum titers[18]. In addition, prolonged infusion may be valuable to maintain the circulating gamma-interferon activity. Toxicities have included fever, chills, fatigue and anorexia similar to that seen with alpha- and beta-interferon. Dose-limiting hypotension was apparent at 60 million units/m^2. When compared to previous studies with alpha-interferon, antiviral titers were generally lower and more transiently maintained with gamma-interferon. In these early studies, striking immunomodulation of NK and monocyte activity was not aparent. An antiproliferative effect on lymphocytes was seen but no antitumor activity in this initial trial was observed. Considerable lot-to-lot variation in the biological activity was noted and this observation emphasizes the need to pursue biological pharmaceuticals of high purity in the absence of other contaminating substances if one is to understand the biological effects of a particular lymphokine or cytokine.

The broader immunomodulatory activity of gamma-interferon and the reported higher antiproliferative activity of this interferon in comparison to alpha- or beta-interferon is of interest. In addition, reports have emphasized the synergistic capability of alpha- or beta-interferon when added to gamma-interferon[19]. These preliminary reports will need to be confirmed by more extensive preclinical trials and the exploitation of these effects in clinical trials is anticipated.

INTERLEUKIN-2 (IL-2)

IL-2 was originally described as a biological activity of stimulated lymphocytes which supported the growth of certain T cells bearing the IL-2 receptor[20]. Subsequent generation of IL-2 from stimulated cell lines and finally the cloning of IL-2 has made available large quantities of purified material for preclinical and clinical trials[21]. A model for the activity of IL-2 is illustrated in Fig. 1 and its biochemical and biological

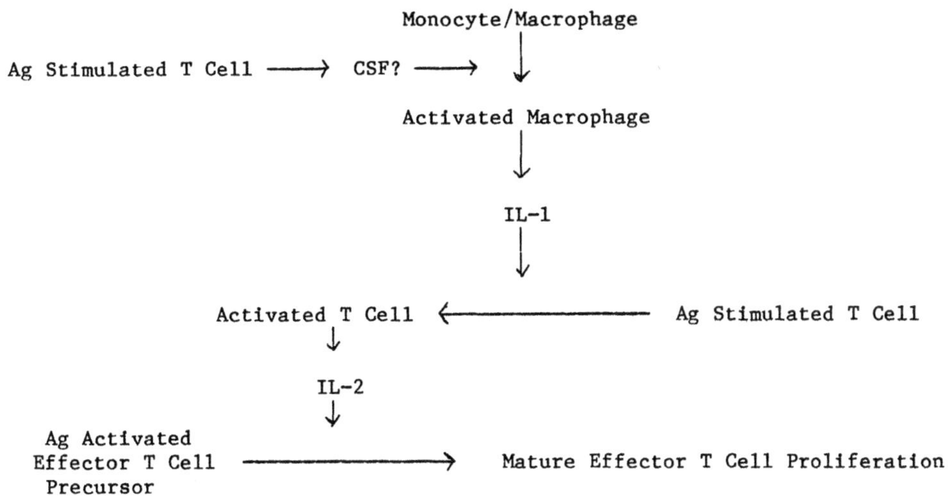

Fig. 1. Interleukin Stimulation of Cellular Immume Response

properties are outlined in Table 7. IL-2 has been utilized to support the proliferation of T-effector cells in vitro in the hope that large quantities of these effector cells can be utilized therapeutically after expansion to sufficient numbers[22,23]. There have been attempts to directly infuse IL-2 to stimulate T-cell proliferation in vivo and/or to correct a T-cell defect in vivo[23,24]. Acquired immunodeficiency symdrome (AIDS) represents a clinical model where IL-2 may be useful. Patients with this syndrome have a selective defect in T-helper cells and a reversal of the T-helper/suppressor ratio in addition to certain other immunological deficiencies which may underlie their susceptibility to multiple infections and may also contribute to the development of Kaposi's sarcoma and lymphoma which is increasingly seen in this patient population. There is preliminary evidence that IL-2 partially corrects the T-cell defect when AIDS patient's T cells are coincubated with this biological in vitro[25]. Similar findings in other immunodeficiencies have been reported[26].

Table 7. Properties of Human IL-2

Biochemical Properties[a]		Biological Properties
1. Sensitivity to Treatments		1. Origin
a. Boiling	+	a. Mature helper T-cells
b. RNAase, DNAase	-	b. Macrophages required
c. Trypsin	+	c. Antigen/mitogen required
d. Freezing	-	2. Target Cell
e. N-ethylmaleimide	-	a. Any activated T-cell
f. Dithiothreitol	-	b. Resting T-cell inactive
g. Hg Cl2	-	c. NK cells
2. Stabilized by:		3. Biological Effect
a. polyethylene gylcol	+	a. Binds to specific receptor
b. albumin	+	b. Promotes entry into S phase
c. glycerol	-	c. Stimulates proliferation
3. Mol. Wt. (SDS-PAGE)	12-13,000	4. Specifies Specificity
4. Isoelectric point	6.8	a. Very little; active in other primates, cow, cats, rodents

[a] Purified IL-2 stabilized with polyethylene glycol was used.

Adapted from Russetti, F. - BRMP Lymphokine Retreat

Preliminary clinical trials administering IL-2 to patients with AIDS have also shown some encouraging results with respect to correcting this defect.

MONOCLONAL ANTIBODIES

The therapeutic use of murine-derived monoclonal antibodies in early phase I trials in humans has been reviewed[7,27]. It is important to confirm that antibodies, when given i.v., actually reach the tumor cells and show a degree of specificity. While radioisotope-labedled antibodies can be used to image the tumor, sensitive immunological techniques, such as immunoperoxidase and flow cytometry, provide direct evidence for localization of the antibody on the tumor cell membrane. In this regard, patients with malignant melanoma represents a unique population because of the accessibility of their cutaneous tumor nodules for biopsy. The 9.2.27 antimelanoma monoclonal antibody was selected since it recognizes a melanoma-associated antigen (250,000 dalton chondroitin sulfate proteoglycan core glycoprotein) on most (90%) melanomas and is relatively selective for the tumor cells[8]. We have also conducted a phase I study in chronic lymphocytic leukemia (CLL) and cutaneous T-cell lymphomas (CCL) with T101 monocloncal antibody[9]. T101 binds to a 65,000 dalton antigen, found on circulating normal T lymphocytes, malignant T lymphocytes, and B-cell-derived chronic lymphocytic leukemia cells.

IN VIVO LOCALIZATION OF MONOCLONAL ANTIBODY IN MELANOMA

These initial studies were designed to focus primarily on antibody localization on tumor cells and the immunologic response to murine monoclonal antibody. Eight patients with malignant melanoma whose tumors reacted *in vitro* with the 9.2.27 monoclonal antibody were treated with escalating doses of antibody to demonstrate localization of antibody in skin nodules as determined by repeated biopsies after treatment. All patients were monitored for clinical response and toxicity, antibody pharmacokinetics, antigenic modulation, and anti-murine antibody formation.

Biopsies were performed from 1 to 4 days following infusion of 9.2.27. Antibody was routinely detected by immunohistology in subcutaneous skin lesions following dosages above 10 mg. Localization was related to quantity of antibody infused as the intensity and homogeneity of tumor staining increased with increasing dose. In addition, the diffusion of antibody out into the tumor nodule was clearly dose dependent. *In vivo* localization of monoclonal antibody in subcutaneous tumors was detected in 6 of 8 patients and the flow cytometry data generally correlated with the immunoperoxidase data (Table 8). Flow cytometry also

Table 8. In Vitro and In Vivo Reactivity of 9.2.27 antibody with melanoma cells in cutaneous skin lesions

Patient	Dose 9.2.27	Days Post Treatment	Flow Cytometry (%) In Vitro	Flow Cytometry (%) In Vivo	Immunoperoxidase† In Vitro	Immunoperoxidase† In Vivo
BF	Pretreatment		83	ND	++	-
	1 mg	1	0	0	+	-
	50 mg	1	72	0	++	+
	200 mg	1	ND	ND	++	+
MF	Pretreatment		97	ND	++	-
	10 mg	1	98	2	+	-
	100 mg	1	72	50	+	+
	200 mg	4	98	91	+	+
CS	Pretreatment		76	ND	++	-
	1 mg	1	91	0	++	-
	200 mg	1	41	35	++	+

demonstrated that there was no antigenic modulation secondary to therapy. It was clear that the tumor cells were not saturated with the 9.2.27 antibody _in vivo_ even after the 200 mg dose since a greater intensity of staining was observed when excess 9.2.27 was added _in vitro_.

IN VIVO LOCALIZATION OF T101 ANTIBODY AND ANTIGENIC MODULATION OF THE T65 ANTIGEN

Thirteen patients with stage IV chronic lymphocytic leukemia were treated. _In vivo_ binding of T101 to circulating leukemia cells was demonstrated in all patients treated. We compared _in vivo_ versus _in vitro_ staining in one representative patient from each treatment group (Figure 2). In the lower curves, only fluorescein-labeled goat anti-mouse immunoglobulin was added to the cells (_in vivo_ labeling). Excess T101 antibody was added to the same cell specimens (upper curve), followed by the fluorescein-labeled secondary antibody, to determine the percent labeling of cells _in vitro_. At 1 mg, a small proportion (25%) of circulating cells was stained _in vivo_ while excess antibody

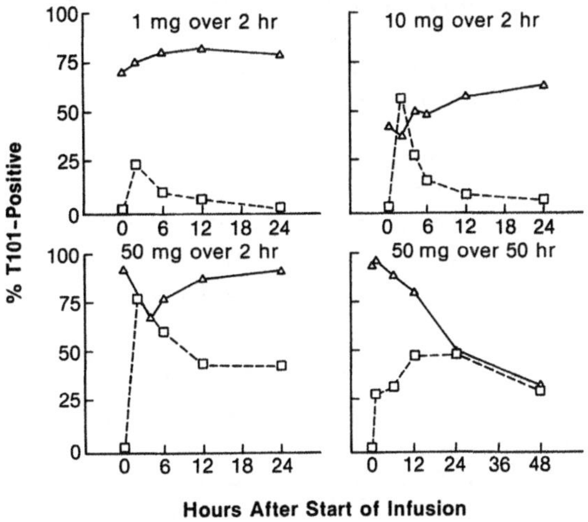

Fig. 2. In vivo versus in vitro binding of T101 antibody by circulating chronic lymphocytic leukemia cells.

stained 80% of the cells _in vitro_. Immediately following a 2-hour infusion of 10 mg of antibody, there was a maximum number of _in vivo_ stained circulating cells, which equaled the number stained _in vitro_. This rapidly declined over the next few hours as T101 was lost from the cell surface membrane or these cells were removed from the circulation. Following a rapid infusion of 40 mg of T101 there was again maximum _in vivo_ binding of T101 to circulating cells immediately following therapy.

In contrast to the results obtained following 10 mg infusions over 2 hours, prolonged infusions of 50 and 100 mg of T101 monoclonal antibody (1 to 2 mg/hour) resulted in nearly 100% modulation of the T65 antigen, secondary to this prolonged infusion, preventing binding of T101 antibody to the cell surface membrane. This modulation was maintained throughout the infusion and prevented any signficant reduction of the circulating cell count. Bone marrow and circulating cells recovered most of their T65 antigen expression by 24 hours after therapy.

Bone marrow samples were removed to determine _in vivo_ localization of T101 antibody in leukemic bone marrow cells. Prior to therapy, 90% of the cells stained _in vitro_ with T101 antibody. Eighty-one percent of the leukemic bone marrow cells were labeled _in vivo_ 2 hours after infusion of 10 mg of T101, with only 10% additional labeling when excess T101 was added _in vitro_. In addition, antigenic modulation was demonstrated in 1 patient's bone marrow tumor cell population 2 hours after the 10 mg infusion of T101. Twenty-four hours after therapy, the bone marrow cells no longer had in-vivo-bound T101 on the cell surface membrane and the cells had fully recovered expression of the T65 antigen.

Lymph nodes were removed from 1 patient 5 hours after a 2-hour infusion of 10 mg of T101 and from another patient at the completion of a 50-hour infusion of 50 mg of antibody. In neither case could we detect in vivo labeling of tumor cells or antigenic modulation of CLL cells in the lymph node, while in both cases greater than 70% of the cells stained with T101 in vitro. These data strongly suggest that T01 did not reach the lymph node and did not label lymph node cells in vivo. This was not surprising as we could not detect circulating free T101 in these patients' serum. In order to increase the amount of free T101 in the serum, 1 patient was treated with a 50-mg infusion of T101 over 50 hours to modulate his circulating and bone marrow leukemia cells. Immediately following this therapy, the patient was given 5, 10, 50, and 100 mg of T101 antibody, each by infusion over 1 hour. Therapy was stopped due to hypotension 15 minutes (25 mg) into the 100-mg dose of T101. At this point, 5.4 ug/ml of free T101 was measured in the patient's serum. A lymph node biopsy 1 hour after the completion of these infusions therapy demonstrated nearly 100% modulation of lymph node cells. These cells were cultued in vitro without T101, and after 5 days 83% of the cells expressed the T65 antigen. These data strongly suggest that T101 reached these lymph node cells in vivo and induced antigenic modulation.

PHARMACOKINETICS AND ANTIGLOBULIN RESPONSE

To assess the circulating levels of murine monoclonal antibody, serum of patients was assayed beginning with the end of infusion and 3 and 24 hours post infusion. Peak values of 9.2.27 progressively increased wih escalating doses. Circulating antibody levels were dose related. Higher and more prolonged levels of 9.2.27 were achieved with higher doses of antibody. Further tests indicated that circulating 9.2.27 was not complexed with antiglobulin and could still bind to cultured melanoma cells.

The transient antiglobulin response did not impede localization of 9.2.27 in cutaneous nodules as there was an increment in the amount of bound antibody in nodules biopsied following the 100 and 200 mg doses. Three of 8 patients had measurable increases in antiglobulin responses (either of the IgG or IgM) after administration of the 10 or 50 mg doses and a loss of demonstrable antiglobulin at the higher dose levels. In the other 5 patients there was no change in antiglobulin activity from baseline levels at any dose level of 9.2.27.

Serum specimens from patients receiving T101 were quantitated for human IgG, IgM, or IgA anti-T101 titers using an ELISA. While some of the patients demonstrated anti-T101 activity prior to therapy, none of the CLL patients experienced significant increases in anti-T101 activity prior to therapy. None of the CLL patients experienced significant increases in anti-T101 titer over the period of the study. Further experiments revealed that the anti-T101 activity detected in both patient and normal control specimen was not specific for either the T101 antibody or mouse IgG_{2a} molecules in that similar degrees of reactivity were observed using IgG preparations of rabbit, rat, guinea pig, or goat origin.

Measureable quantities of circulating mouse IgG (T101) were not detected in patients receiving less than 100 mg dose levels. The detection limit for the assay employed was in the range of 0.2 to 0.4 ug/ml. Both patients receiving 100 mg doses of T101 over 50-hour priods of infusion demonstrated measurable levels of circulating mouse IgG. In both patients, detectable circulating levels of muring IgG were not obtained until 24 hours after starting the first infusion, reaching maximal concentrations of 1.0 and 3.5 ug/ml, respectively. Following modulation (third infusion of 100 mg), circulating murine IgG was detected in 2 patients immediately prior to initiating the third dose and rose to levels of 4.2 and 5 ug/ml over the period of infusion.

CLINICAL RESPONSE

There were no measurable decreases in the size of the melanoma skin lesions, lymph nodes, or visceral metastases during treatment with 9.2.27, although some of the nodules softened in 2 patients.

In patients treated with T101, circulating leukemia cell counts routinely dropped to approximately 50% of pretreatment levels immediately following a 2-hour infusion. However, by 24 to 48 hours the cell count rapidly recovered to the pretreatment level. Two of the patients treated with a 2-hour infusion of 10 mg maintained a reduction in their circulating leukemic cell count to the pretreatment levels throughout the course of therapy. Response in patients treated with prolonged infusions of antibody was quite different. These patients demonstrated a 20% to 50% drop immediately following the infusion of monclonal antibody that reached its nadir approximately 12 to 24 hours into the infusion (25 to 50 mg of antibody administered). Cell counts gradually rose over the next hours, and by the time the infusion was completed, cell counts had recovered to pretreatment levels in most patients. The circulating cell count correlated inversely with the degree of antigenic modulation of the T65 antigen. None of the patients demonstrated a reduction in the size of lymph nodes or organs or showed an improvement in platelets or red blood cell counts. Localization of T101 in the skin lesions with some improvement in the skin of CTCL patients was seen[9].

CONCLUSIONS

The use of biologicals and biological response modifiers represents the emerging fourth modality of cancer treatment[13]. In addition, these agents and this technology have far broader applications than cancer therapeutics. Given the large number of cloned biologicals and the virtually unlimited numbr of recombinant molecules which can be produced therfrom, along with the great variety of monoclonal antibodies that can be produced through hybridoma technology, it is apparent that the coming decade will produce new challenges for those involved in developing new anticancer therapies[28]. Over the past 30 years, only approximately 40 chemotherapeutic agents of the 500,000 tested have cleared all of the preclinical evluations and been made available for standard clinical use. By contrast, it now appears that we will have a comparatively large number of new, potentially useful therapeutic biologicals available within the next decade[29]. This tremendous expansion of agents and approaches available for cancer theapeutics will increase our opportunities and amplify our problems with the preclinical evaluation of these agents and their translation to the clinic. New mechanisms for the testing of these biologicals and the selection of the "most likely to succeed" need to be developed. Additionally, current methods used by pharmaceutical manufacturers and the regulations established by Federal agencies will be inhibitory in the face of a large number of biologicals to be tested. The development of novel approaches will be necessary if these biologicals are to be effectively and rapidly made available for clinical trials[28].

A new era has begun. Immunomodulators, lymphokines/cytokines, and monoclonal antibodie are being extensively evaluated in preclinical models and in clinical studies. Historically, the chemical, bacterial, and viral immunomoduators have not proven highly useful in clinical trials[30]. By contrast, it is already apparent that alpha-interferon has evident antitumor effects even in certain patients with bulky disease[12]. This finding should give pause to those believing the immunological dogma that these agents can only be active in minimal residual disase. Like chemotherapy and radiotheapy, biologicals and biological response modifiers may be more active with lesser tumor burdens; but the early data indicates that activity and hence selection of compound for further study can be assessed in patients with advanced disease.

A very clear demonstration that monoclonal antibody, when administered i.v., can selectively locate on the tumor cell membrane gives strong support to the concept that these agents may be useful in specific targeting of cancer therapy. Already, investigations into the use of immunoconjugates are indicating that monoclonal antibodies can be used to carry drugs, toxins,and radioisotopes to the cancer cell with a specificity heretofore unavailable in cancer therapeutics.

We have reached a plateau in cancer treatment utilizing the three classic modalities of surgery, radiotherapy, and chemotherapy. The advent of biologicals and biological response modifiers as the fourth modality of cancer treatment is serving to make available new and more selective therapeutic approaches to the treatment of cancer[13].

REFERENCES

1. Fidler,I.J., Berendt, m., and Oldham, R.K., J. Biol. Resp. Modif., (in press) (1982).
2. Talmadge, J.E., Oldham, R.K., and Fidler, I.J., J. Biol. Resp. Modif., (in press) (1983).
3. Smalley, R.v., Talmade, J., Oldham, R.K., and Thurman, G.B., in Byrom, N.A., and Hobbs, J.R., eds., Thymic Factor Therapy, London: Academic Press, (in press) (1983).
4. Talmadege, J.E., Fidler, I.J., and Oldham, R.K., in Spitzy, K.H. and Karrer, K., eds., Proceedings of the 13th International Chemotherapy Congress, Vienna, Austria, (1983).
5. Talmadge, J.E., Uithoven, K.A., Lenz, B.F., and Chirigos, M.A., (Manuscript Submitted) (1983).
6. Talmadge, J.E., Lenz, B.F., Collin, M.S., et al., in Spitzy, K.H. and Karrer, K., eds., Proceedings of the 13th International Chemotherapy Congress, Vienna, Austria, (1983).
7. Oldham, R.K., J. Clin. Oncol. 1:582 (1983).
8. Oldham, R.K., Morgan, A.C., Woodhouse, C.S., Schroff, R.W., Abrams, P.G., and Foon, K.A., Med. Oncol. Tumor Pharmacother., (in press) (1984).
9. Foon, K.A., Bunn, P.A., Schroff, R.W., et al, in Langman, R.E., Trowbridge, I.S., and Dulbecco, R., eds., Monocloncal Antibodies and Cancer, New York: Academic Press (in press) (1983).

10. Smalley, R.V., and Oldham, R.K., J. Biol. Resp. Modif., 5:40 1 (1983).
11. Herberman, R.B., and Thurman, G.B., J. Biol. Resp. Modif. (in press) (1983).
12. Oldham, R.K., in Zoon, K.C., and Liu, D., Proceeding of Workshop on Interferon, New York: Elsevier (in press) (1983).
13. Oldham, R.K., Cancer Treat. Rpt., (in press) (1983).
14. Thurman, G.B., Brande, I.A., Gray, P.W., Stevenson, H.C., and Oldham, R.K., (Manuscript submitted) (1983).
15. Schreiber, R.D., Pace, J.L., Russell, S.W., Altman, A., and Katz, D.H., J. Immunol., 131:826 (1983).
16. Gemsa, D., Debatin, K.L., Kramer, W., et al., J. Immunol. 131:833
17. Zlotnik, A., Roberts, W.K., Vasil, A., et al., J. Immunol. 131:794 (1983).
18. Oldham, R.K., Sherwin, S.A., Maluish, A., Long, C.W., Watson, T., and Foon, K.A., in Goldstein, A.L., ed., Thymic Hormones and Lymphokines, New York: Plenum Press (in press) (1983).
19. Fleischman, Jr., W.R., Cancer Res. 42:869 (1982).
20. Ruscetti, F.W., Morgan, D.A., and Gallo, R.C., J. Immunol. 119:131 (1977).
21. Gillis, S., J. Clin. Immunol. 3(1):1 (1983).
22. Cheever, M.A., Greenberg, P.D., and Fefer, A., J. Immunol. 126:1318.
23. Cheever, M.A., Greenbeg, P.D., Fefer, A., and Gillis, S, J.Exp. Med. 155:968 (1982).
24. Donohue, J.H., and Rosenberg, S.A., J. Immunol. 130:2203 (1983).
25. Palladino, M.A., Welte, K., Ciobanu, N., Mertelsmann, R., and Oetgen, H.F., in proceedings from the Converence on Thymic Hormones and Lymphokines, May 31-June 3, Washington, D.C., p. 79 (1983).
26. Flomenberg, N., Welte, K., Mertelsmann, R., et al, J. Immunol. 130:2644 (1983).
27. Ritz, J., and Schlossman, S.F., Blood 59:1 (1982).
28. Oldham, R.K., J. Biol. Resp. Modif. 2:199 (1983).
29. Oldham, R.K., J.N.C.I. 70:789 (1983).
30. Oldham, R.K., and Smalley, R.V., J. Biol. Resp. Modif. 2:1 (1983).

INDEX

GPSR Compliance

The European Union's (EU) General Product Safety Regulation (GPSR) is a set of rules that requires consumer products to be safe and our obligations to ensure this.

If you have any concerns about our products, you can contact us on ProductSafety@springernature.com

In case Publisher is established outside the EU, the EU authorized representative is:

Springer Nature Customer Service Center GmbH
Europaplatz 3
69115 Heidelberg, Germany

Batch number: 10615115

Printed by Printforce, the Netherlands